The Plateau-proof Diet™

for

Hypertension

(Essential [idiopathic] high blood pressure)

George M. Ekema

Edited by Marjet D. Heitzer

GƏV PITTSBURGH

Published by G&V PITTSBURGH
A division of G&V Publishing, Inc.

Printed in the United States of America

ISBN 0-9768150-7-9

Dedicated to improving the quality of human life by
providing the cutting edge in weight loss science

For questions, comments, and a free subscription to *Trimming America*™ (The Journal of The Plateau-proof Diet Foundation),

logon to

www.plateauproofdiet.com

Contents

Introduction ▫━▫━▫━▫ **7**

------*Chapter One*------
Metabolism in Normal Health and in Hypertension ▫━▫━▫ **13**

- *Introduction to carbohydrates* ▫━▫━▫ 14

- *Introduction to fats* ▫━▫━▫▫━▫━▫ 15

- *Introduction to proteins* ▫━▫━▫━▫ 17

- *Metabolism* ▫━▫━▫━▫▫━▫━▫ 18

- *Carbohydrate metabolism* ▫━▫━▫ 19

- *Carbohydrates and hypertension* ▫━▫━▫━▫ 20

- *Fat metabolism* ▫━▫━▫━▫▫━▫━▫ 23

- *Fat and hypertension* ▫━▫━▫━▫ 24

- *Protein metabolism* ▫━▫━▫━▫ 27

- *Protein and hypertension* ▫━▫━▫━▫ 28

- *Metabolism summary and discussion* ▫━▫ 30

- *Summary of metabolism in hypertension* □■□■□■□ 33

------Chapter Two------

The Fundamentals of Obesity and Weight loss □□■□■□■□ **35**

- *Obesity* □■□■□□■□■□ 36

- *What causes obesity?* □■□■□□■□■□□■□■□ 36

- *Are there any health risks associated with obesity?* □■□■□ 38

- *How is obesity measured?* □■□■□□■□■□ 38

- *The waist-to-hip ratio* □■□■□□■□■□ 39

- *Obesity and hypertension* □■□■□■□ 40

- *Confused by the many diets and dieting terminology?* □■□ 41

- *Types of weight loss diets* □■□■□□■□■□ 42

- *Why is the plateau-proof diet superior to all of these weight loss diets?* □■□■□□■□■□□■□■□ 44

------Chapter Three------

Popular weight loss diets – where we were before the Plateau-proof Diet □■□□■□■□□■□■□□■□■□ **46**

- *Low-carb, very low-carb, and low-fat diets* □■□■□■□ 48

- *Discussion on low-carb and low-fat diets* □■□■□■□ 64

- *Are low-carb diets safe?* ▫▬▫▬▫▬▫▫▬▫▬▫▬▫ 67

- *Are low-carb and low-fat diets effective treatments*

  for obesity? ▫▬▫▬▫▬▫▫▬▫▬▫▬▫▫▬▫▬▫ 68

- *High-protein or high-fat* ▫▬▫▬▫▬▫▫▬▫▬▫ 69

- *High-fiber and low glycemic load diets* ▫▬▫▬▫▬▫ 71

------Chapter Four------
The Plateau-proof Diet™ **for Hypertension – Reversing the symptoms of hypertension with an efficient and sustainable weight loss** ▬▫▬▫ **73**

- *The science behind the plateau-proof diet* ▫▬▫▬▫▬▫ 73

- *The logic behind the food tables – how the plateau-proof diet works, and why it is the best weight loss diet by a vast margin* ▫▬▫▬▫▬▫▫▬▫▬▫▬▫ 77

- *The CP and FP formulas* ▫▬▫▬▫▬▫▫▬▫▬▫▬▫ 79

- *Derivation of the CP formula* ▫▬▫▬▫▬▫▫▬▫▬▫▬▫ 81

- *Derivation of the FP formula* ▫▬▫▬▫▬▫▫▬▫▬▫▬▫ 85

- *How cutoff values of CP and FP were determined* ▫▬▫▬▫ 87

- *How to use the plateau-proof diet* ▫▬▫▬▫▬▫▫▬▫▬▫▬▫ 88

- *Weight loss profile of the plateau-proof diet* ▫▬▫▬▫▬▫ 91

- *'Green' Rotation One Table* 92

- *'Yellow' Rotation One Table* 97

- *'Red' Rotation One Table* 100

- *'Green' Rotation Two Table* 112

- *'Yellow' Rotation Two Table* 117

- *'Red' Rotation Two Table* 121

------Chapter Five------

The Plateau-proof Diet™ Turbo for Hypertension – The weight loss solution for stubborn obesity 132

- *Turbo 'Green' Rotation One Table* 134

- *Turbo 'Yellow' Rotation One Table* 139

- *Turbo 'Red' Rotation One Table* 141

- *Turbo 'Green' Rotation Two Table* 154

- *Turbo 'Yellow' Rotation Two Table* 159

- *Turbo 'Red' Rotation Two Table* 163

------*Chapter Six*------

Weight Loss Dieting in Hypertension – facts and fiction □—□ 174

- *Can dietary supplements affect weight loss?* □—□ 174

- *Does decreasing the amount of iron in the diet affect weight loss?* □—□ 177

- *Does increasing the amount of fruits and vegetable in the diet affect weight loss?* □—□—□□—□ 177

- *Are there foods that promote weight loss?* □—□—□ 178

- *Weight loss from cocoa powder?* □—□—□ 178

- *Does increasing calcium intake from dairy affect weight loss?* □—□—□—□□—□—□—□□—□—□—□ 179

- *Does alcohol have a role in obesity and weight loss?* □—□ 179

Appendix I – Weight / height charts for measuring obesity □—□ **181**

Appendix II – Sample 400 g (14.1 oz) meals □—□—□ **184**

Bibliography □—□—□—□□—□—□—□□—□—□—□□—□—□—□□—□ **186**

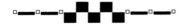

Introduction

Hypertension means high blood pressure. A person is considered to have hypertension if systolic blood pressure is consistently over 140 mmHg and/or diastolic blood pressure is consistently over 90 mmHg. A person is considered to have pre-hypertension if systolic blood pressure is consistently between 120 mmHg and 139 mmHg, and/or diastolic blood pressure is consistently between 80 mmHg and 89 mmHg. Hypertension that has no identifiable cause is called idiopathic hypertension or essential hypertension. Secondary hypertension refers to hypertension that is caused by another condition. Some of the causes of secondary hypertension include; adrenal gland tumors, Cushing's syndrome, kidney disease, hemolytic-uremic syndrome, Henoch-Schonlein purpura, periarteritis nodosa, radiation enteritis, retroperitoneal fibrosis, and Wilm's tumor.

Idiopathic hypertension accounts for the absolute majority of the cases of hypertension. The Plateau-proof Diet for Hypertension is designed for weight loss in idiopathic hypertension only, and is not recommended for secondary hypertension. Patients should consult with their primary health care provider before starting this diet or any other weight loss diet. While on this diet, patients are advised to restrict their sodium intake (from salt, MSG, baking soda, etc) to less than 1.5 grams per day (equivalent to half a teaspoon of table salt). Sodium intake can be significantly reduced by avoiding packaged foods and restaurant foods.

If not properly controlled, idiopathic hypertension may result in severe conditions such as; heart disease, blood vessel damage, kidney disease, stroke, vision loss, and brain damage. It has been shown that controlling idiopathic hypertension with drugs alone may not eliminate the risk of developing some of these conditions. This is one of the important reasons why overweight and obese patients should consider dietary therapy as part of a lifestyle change that includes moderate exercise. Diets such as the DASH diet and the Mediterranean diet have been shown to be effective for controlling blood pressure. These diets are limited; however, by their inability to affect weight loss in patients with idiopathic hypertension.

It has been shown that most cases of idiopathic hypertension can be reversed by weight loss, and even modest weight loss can affect a significant decrease in blood pressure. Most individuals with idiopathic hypertension are either overweight or obese. It is more difficult for individuals with idiopathic hypertension to lose weight compared to normotensive (free of hypertension) individuals of the same weight and body profile. Idiopathic hypertension is characterized by deficiencies in carbohydrate and fat metabolism. It has been demonstrated that idiopathic hypertension, per se, is an insulin-resistant state. Most cases of hypertension are therefore characterized by glucose-intolerance as in type II diabetes mellitus. It has also been demonstrated that there are significant alterations in fat metabolism in idiopathic hypertension. It is now known that these alterations in fat metabolism may begin in childhood, and that they precede the symptoms of hypertension and alterations in carbohydrate metabolism.

The Plateau-proof Diet for Hypertension takes advantage of these peculiarities of macronutrient metabolism in idiopathic hypertension to ease the difficulty in attaining and sustaining weight loss that is characteristic of idiopathic hypertension. The ultimate purpose of the diet is to affect a sustainable weight loss that may lead to a reversal of the symptoms of idiopathic hypertension. The Plateau-proof Diet for Hypertension is not intended to replace your current drug treatment for hypertension, and you should consult your primary health care provider before and during this weight loss diet therapy.

The high incidence of idiopathic hypertension in the United States is corroborated by the high incidence of obesity. The National Institutes of Health (NIH) estimates that 129.6 million adults (64.5%) are overweight. 61.3 million adults (30.5%) are obese. Only 33.5% of adult Americans are at a healthy weight. The NIH also estimates that 15.3% of children and 15.5% of adolescents are overweight. Apart from making America look big, obesity is making America ill. Obesity has been linked to a number of diseases, including; heart disease, stroke, diabetes, high blood pressure, gout, sleep apnea (and other breathing disorders), osteoarthritis, gall bladder disease, gall stones, emotional disorders, colon cancer, rectal cancer, prostate cancer, ovarian cancer, cervical cancer, uterine cancer, breast cancer, cancer of the gall bladder, etc. Morbidity from obesity is high, and a slightly obese individual is twice as likely as a non-obese individual to die prematurely. Costing America $117 billion per year in health care, obesity is overdue a sustainable treatment.

Although proper dieting is the most promising means of controlling obesity and consequently idiopathic hypertension, weight loss diets have so far fallen short. Most weight loss diets available today are capable of affecting an initial weight loss. Weight loss with all of these diets; however, stops prematurely (the plateau), and no further weight loss is possible even with further restrictions of the diet. The weight loss plateau is the point where weight loss stops prematurely regardless of the dieter's efforts. The weight loss plateau is usually followed by a relapse into weight gain. Everyone who has been on a weight loss diet is familiar with the weight loss plateau. The weight loss diets available today fail to affect a complete weight loss because of two important reasons – they are one-dimensional and static. Obesity is a complicated, multidimensional, and dynamic condition. In order for a weight loss diet to be effective in reversing obesity, it has to be multidimensional and dynamic – these are the minimum essential requirements. None of the weight loss diets available today come close to meeting these minimum essential requirements. The plateau-proof diet is a multidimensional and dynamic weight loss diet that is up to the task of controlling obesity in America and the rest of the world. It is a just claim that the plateau-proof diet is the best weight loss diet by a vast margin.

The plateau-proof diet is a reflection of the state-of-the-art in biomedical and clinical research in idiopathic hypertension, obesity, and weight loss. Weight loss is largely a matter of manipulation of the three macronutrients; carbohydrate, fat, and protein. Many popular weight loss diets merely decrease the amount of one macronutrient, for example the low-carb and low-fat diets. Other weight loss diets are dependent on the archaic notion of counting calories. The plateau-proof diet takes into consideration all of the macronutrients and their caloric contribution, amongst other things. Using the state-of-the-art in scientific knowledge, the plateau-proof diet is based on two simple mathematical formulas. The formulas have been used to assign indices (numbers) to a large selection of foods. These foods have been placed in 'green', 'yellow', and 'red' tables. The smaller the number assigned to a food, the better that food is for weight loss. Foods with the smallest numbers are in the 'green' tables, while foods with the largest numbers are in the 'red' tables. The 'yellow' tables are intermediate, and these foods are used mainly for weight maintenance following weight loss from foods in the 'green' tables.

The plateau-proof diet is easy to use, simply amounting to comparing the 'green' and 'yellow' tables with your grocery list. There is no counting of calories with this diet, since the absolute caloric contribution of each macronutrient is already considered in the mathematical formulas that created the tables. By providing a large number and variety of foods to choose from, the diet is less stressful and more sustainable than other weight loss diets. The diet is also controllable, allowing the dieter to lose weight rapidly or slowly. The diet provides two 'green' tables and two 'yellow' tables, and requires a rotation between them. This rotation makes the diet dynamic and minimizes the chances of the weight loss plateau.

The Plateau-proof Diet for Hypertension is presented in Chapter four, and The Plateau-proof Diet Turbo for Hypertension (a more restrictive adaptation for stubborn obesity) is presented in Chapter five. Chapters one through three provide background information that is important in understanding the mechanisms behind The Plateau-proof Diet. Although it is not required to understand the mechanisms of the diet, dieters who understand the fundamental principles behind The Plateau-proof Diet are likely to have more success than other dieters. The fundamental principles behind The Plateau-proof Diet are not complicated, and everyone is encouraged to make an effort in understanding them completely. Remember that you can always bring your questions and comments to www.plateauproofdiet.com.

The Plateau-proof Diet for Hypertension is not intended to be a replacement of your current treatment for idiopathic hypertension. Please consult with your primary health care provider before starting this or any other weight loss diet.

Metabolism in Normal Health and in Hypertension

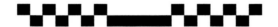

What happens to the foods we eat when they get into the body? All the foods we eat are mainly composed of the three macronutrients; carbohydrates (carbs), fats, and proteins. What happens to these macronutrients when they get into the body is called metabolism. It is important to know the basic metabolism of carbs, fats and proteins for 3 reasons:

1) To understand the basic principles behind the plateau-proof diet. The plateau-proof diet is easy to follow, having been simplified into a few tables; however, it is beneficial for dieters to understand the basic principles behind this diet. Although everyone will benefit from the efficiency of this diet, the dieters who understand the basic principles behind this diet are likely to enjoy greater success.

2) Weight gain and weight loss are dependent on proportions of carbohydrates, fats and proteins in the diet; with emphasis on their fates as determined by metabolism (and other factors that will be discussed later). Understanding the basics of metabolism will give the dieter an appreciation for the important physiological changes that occur in the body during weight gain and weight loss. This knowledge is beneficial for the management of weight loss in hypertension.

3) There are significant changes in the metabolism of two of the macronutrients (carbohydrate and fat) in hypertension[1-92]. The majority of hypertension cases are due to excess body weight[23,93-99]. The deficiencies in metabolism and symptoms of hypertension may be reversed with relatively modest and proper weight loss[94,96-98,100,101]. Due to the metabolic deficiencies; however, diet-induced weight loss in hypertension is complicated and dangerous if misguided. It is beneficial therefore to understand both normal metabolism and metabolism during hypertension, in order to have control of the efficacy and safety of both your weight loss diet and your weight maintenance diet.

This chapter covers the basic metabolism of carbohydrates, fats and proteins. It goes into just as much detail as is required to appreciate your body and what the plateau-proof diet is about to do to it.

Introduction to carbohydrates

Carbohydrates are the main energy source for the healthy body, and are classified as either glycemic or non-glycemic. Glycemic carbohydrates provide energy to the body as sugar upon digestion and absorption into the blood stream. Non-glycemic carbohydrates cannot be digested, and hence do not provide energy to the body (0 calories). There are basically three kinds of carbohydrates – sugars, starch and fiber. Sugars and starch are glycemic carbohydrates, with each gram providing about 4 calories of energy to the body. Starch is essentially a chain of sugars. The role of digestion is to break down this chain into individual simple sugars, because only individual sugars are small enough to cross from the intestine into the blood vessels that line the intestines. The simple sugars include: glucose, fructose and galactose. Glucose is the most abundant. It is also the form into which all carbohydrates are converted for use as fuel in the body. Plant foods such as corn, pasta, cereals and rice are rich in carbohydrates.

Fiber is a non-glycemic carbohydrate, as they provide no energy to the body. The human digestive system does not break down fiber into simple sugars; hence fiber is not an energy source for the body. Fiber is also known as roughage or bulk. Foods such as black-eyed peas, chickpeas, kidney beans and whole-grain cereals are rich in fiber. Since fiber is non-glycemic, an efficient and sustainable weight loss diet should take advantage of this zero calorie bulk. You will see in chapter three that a fiber index is one of the many parameters used in the formulas of the plateau-proof diets.

Introduction to fats

Fats are richer than carbohydrates in calories, with a gram of fat providing 9 calories; more than double the 4 calories provided by a gram of carbohydrate. Just as carbohydrates are made up of chains of sugar, fats are made up of chains of fatty acids. Dietary fat is therefore digested in the intestines and absorbed into the bloodstream as fatty acids. It has been shown in scientific experiments that rapid weight gain and obesity can result from increasing the amount of fat in the diet. It has also been shown that too much fat in the diet may cause other complications that may or may not be related to obesity. These health complications include heart disease, high blood pressure, stroke, cancer, etc. In order to minimize the risk of these diseases, it is recommended that no greater than 30% of dietary calories be derived from fat. While active non-obese individuals may obtain up to 30% of their dietary calories from fat, sedentary and obese individuals should keep this value below 25%. It is also unhealthy to completely eliminate fat from the diet, since it is required for several important physiological processes in our body. In general (not considering special very low-fat dietary plans for weight loss), adults should obtain at least 15% of their energy intake from dietary fats. Pregnant women should increase fat intake to at least 20% in order to provide fatty acids that are required for healthy development of the child in the womb. There are many food sources of fat. We see the obvious fat sources, such as cooking oil and butter, however; a lot of fat is hidden in foods such as snacks, pastries, and packaged foods. There are basically two types of fat – saturated fat and unsaturated fat, distinguished by their chemical structure.

Saturated fats are so defined due to their relatively high hydrogen content. They are mostly derived from animal sources. Meats and whole dairy products such as milk, cream, cheese, butter and ice cream are rich in saturated fat. Saturated fat is also naturally occurring in some plant food sources such as palm kernel oil and coconut oil. Other vegetable oils such as corn oil, soybean oil, and canola oil are naturally unsaturated; however, when they are processed into margarine and vegetable shortening, they become saturated. Additional hydrogen atoms are added to these vegetable oils during processing, making them solid at room temperature. Saturated fat is a significant cause of heart disease and related health problems. It is highly recommended that most dietary fat come from unsaturated fat. Saturated fat should account for less than 20% of total dietary fat.

Unsaturated fats are so defined based on their relatively low hydrogen content. Unsaturated fats are derived from plant (vegetable) sources. Certain vegetable oils such as palm kernel oil and coconut oil are however rich in saturated fats, and must be noted as important exceptions. Unsaturated fats are usually liquid at room temperature. Unsaturated fats do not pose a direct danger to the heart in terms of disease, however; like saturated fat, they provide 9 calories of energy per gram and over-consumption may result is weight gain and possibly obesity.

Introduction to proteins

Protein is made of chains of amino acids, just like carbohydrates are made of chains of sugar. Like carbohydrates and fat, protein can be used as a source of energy for the body. Each gram of protein provides 4 calories of energy. Most of the human body is composed of protein – muscles, blood, skin, hair, etc are mostly protein. Dietary protein is primarily used for building and maintaining the body, and for thousands of other important processes that are required for the body to function. When sufficient energy is not derived from carbohydrates and fats, protein may be used for energy.

The body can make most of the amino acids that are the building blocks of protein. There are a few amino acids that the body cannot make, and these amino acids (known as essential amino acids) must be derived from dietary protein. Dietary proteins derived from animal sources such as fish, meats, eggs and dairy contain all of these essential amino acids, and are referred to as complete proteins. Dietary proteins derived from plant sources such as rice, nuts, beans, etc may be lacking in one or more essential amino acid. Since some sources of animal protein are high in saturated fat, it is a good idea to obtain a significant portion of dietary protein from plant sources and low-fat animal sources such as fish. Since some plant sources don't contain all the essential amino acids, a variety of plant-derived foods must be part of a healthy weight loss diet.

Metabolism

Metabolism is simply the breaking down of glucose, fatty acids, and amino acids into smaller components, or the synthesis (building) of glucose, fatty acids, and amino acids from these smaller components. The breaking down part of metabolism is referred to as catabolism, and the synthesis part is also known as anabolism. Catabolism typically produces energy, while anabolism consumes energy. Metabolism is a dynamic process that takes place in the cells of the body. The direction of metabolism (rate of catabolism versus anabolism) is determined by several factors, most of which are beyond the scope of this book. The most significant determining factor; however, is the abundance and ratio (relative amounts) of glucose, fatty acids and amino acids. Metabolism determines the fate of these nutrients, and therefore provides the logical starting point for the dietary basis of obesity and weight loss.

Carbohydrate metabolism

When carbohydrates are eaten, they are broken down (digested) into glucose, fructose and galactose. Glucose, fructose and galactose are simple sugars that cross into the bloodstream from the intestine. Once these simple sugars are in the bloodstream, they become available for metabolism in the cells of the body. A summary of carbohydrate metabolism is shown in Figure 1. In the first step of carbohydrate metabolism, all three simple sugars are converted to a modified form of glucose called glucose-6-phosphate. Glucose-6-phosphate is broken down into smaller components; pyruvic acid, acetyl CoA, and eventually into carbon dioxide (CO_2) and water (H_2O). The breaking down of glucose into carbon dioxide and water generates the energy that is required by the body to function. When the amount of carbohydrates consumed in the diet exceeds the energy requirements of the body, the excess glucose is stored. Excess glucose is stored in two ways. In the first case, it may be stored as glycogen, a substance that is readily converted back into glucose when the body needs energy. This form of storage is mainly for the short-term, and it is not the preferred form of storage of excess glucose. In the second case, excess glucose is converted to fat and stored in fat cells. Storing excess glucose as fat is more economical for the body, as more calories can be stored in a relatively smaller space.

Under extreme conditions excess glucose may be converted into amino acids. As you will see shortly in the sections on fat and protein metabolism, carbohydrates, fats and proteins can be converted, each into the others, during the course of metabolism. You will also see why this phenomenon is important in the dietary basis of hypertension, obesity, and weight loss.

Carbohydrates and hypertension

The metabolism of carbohydrates takes place inside the cells of the body, as does the metabolism of the other macronutrients. Once carbohydrates are absorbed as glucose into the blood vessels that line the small intestine, the glucose is transported to all the cells of the body via the blood. When the glucose is brought to the proximity of a cell, a hormone called insulin helps the glucose to enter the cell. Insulin is secreted by the pancreas in response to an increase in the level of glucose in the blood. It helps the cells to pick up glucose from blood and convert it into energy. It also facilitates the conversion of excess glucose into glycogen or fat for storage.

It has been adequately demonstrated that idiopathic hypertension is an insulin-resistant state. In hypertension, the cells in the body ignore insulin (insulin resistance)[32,33,35-42,73,102-105]. As a result, glucose in the blood enters the cells at a slower rate, and the levels of glucose in the blood become higher than normal (hyperglycemia). The pancreas responds to the high blood glucose by secreting more insulin (hyperinsulinemia). The more insulin the pancreas secretes, the more the cells in the body become resistant to it. The glucose in the blood is eventually excreted from the body by the kidneys in urine.

Insulin resistance is mainly at the level of muscle cells and fat cells. This defining characteristic of hypertension transforms carbs from a preferred energy source into a potential toxin. Glucose is as bad a toxin as any if its level in the blood is held above normal; as unchecked hyperglycemia will destroy the body rapidly. The metabolism of carbs is clearly compromised in hypertension. The cells pick up glucose at a slower rate than normal, causing the level of glucose in the blood to rise above normal. Dietary intervention in hypertension should compensate for hyperglycemia by substituting refined carbs in the diet for non-glycemic carbs (fiber) and unrefined carbs. These carbs are digested and absorbed into the blood stream slower than refined carbs. Fiber is not digested at all, and does not contribute to blood glucose. Substituting refined carbs with fiber and unrefined carbs is just the beginning of the dietary adjustments in hypertension, regarding carb metabolism and glucose toxicity. The ratio of carbs to the other macronutrients is the key to weight loss dietary intervention in hypertension. Based on the state-of-the-art in biomedical and clinical research, the plateau-proof diet has used simple math formulas to determine which carbs and other macronutrients to eat and which to avoid in hypertension.

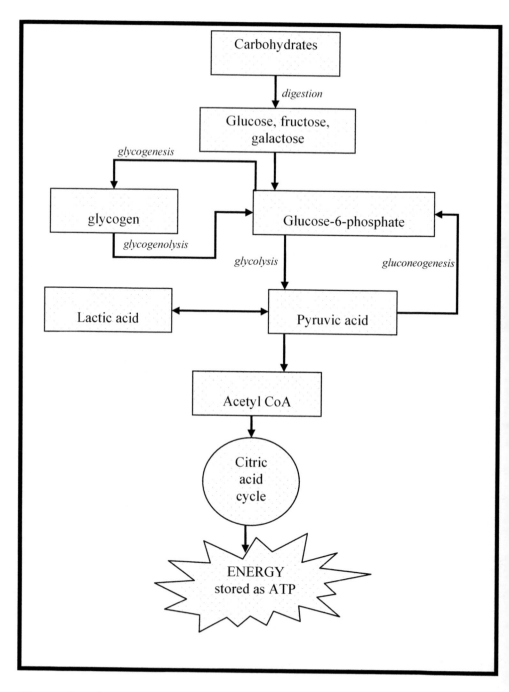

Figure 1 – Summary of carbohydrate metabolism.

Fat metabolism

When fats are eaten, they are broken down (digested) into fatty acids in the intestine. These fatty acids are absorbed into the bloodstream through the blood vessels that line the walls of the intestine. Fatty acids are an important source of energy for the body, with each gram producing more than twice the energy of an equal amount of glucose. A summary of fat metabolism is shown in Figure 2. Except the brain and red blood cells which exclusively use energy from glucose, all parts of the body can use energy from fatty acid metabolism. When fatty acids enter the bloodstream, they can be immediately broken down into acetyl CoA (as is the case with glucose) and eventually to carbon dioxide and water. The breaking down of fatty acids into carbon dioxide and water generates energy for the body. When more fat is consumed in the diet than is required to meet the energy demands of the body, excess fat is stored. Excess fatty acids combine with a molecule called glycerol to form triglycerides. This is the form in which fatty acids are stored in fat cells.

On the other hand, when the total amount of food consumed in the diet provides less energy than is required by the body, some of the fat that is stored in fat cells are broken down to make up for the difference. It may appear from this discussion that weight loss is a matter of simple math – eat less than your body's energy requirement and you will lose weight; eat more than your body's energy requirement and you will gain weight. We will see a little later that obesity and weight loss are more complicated than that; both in normal health and in hypertension. Many weight loss diets focus on this overly simplified view of obesity and weight loss, demanding the meticulous counting of calories. We will see soon enough why this approach to weight loss is flawed and why these diets are ineffective for a sustained weight loss. This is one of the many flaws that are corrected in the plateau-proof diet.

Fat and hypertension

The metabolism of fat is compromised in hypertension[1-11,14,15,19,20,106]. The problem appears to start with visceral (gut) fat cells. More than subcutaneous (under the skin) fat cells, visceral fat cells are particularly dangerous in causing and aggravating the symptoms of hypertension. The visceral fat cells secrete triglycerides (stored fats) more easily than the subcutaneous fat cells. Under normal circumstances, the triglycerides are oxidized (broken down for energy) by cells of the body; mostly by muscle cells. In hypertension, the ability of the muscle cells to oxidize triglycerides is impaired. These cells can pick up triglycerides from the blood, but they can no longer break them down to release energy. The triglycerides accumulate in muscle cells. As the triglyceride accumulation in muscle cells increases, the ability of the cells to respond to insulin decreases (insulin resistance increases)[59,90,107-109]. It was shown in the section on glucose metabolism that an increase in insulin resistance causes an increase in blood glucose levels. We now see that the increase in blood glucose levels is linked to an increase in the level of fat (triglycerides) in the blood. Hypertension is therefore a state of altered carbohydrate and fat metabolism.

The increased secretion of triglycerides in the blood by visceral fat cells is also subject to aggravation from insulin resistance. Under normal circumstances, the secretion of triglycerides by fat cells is controlled by insulin. Insulin instructs these cells to not secrete triglycerides into the blood. When these cells become resistant to insulin, they continue secreting triglycerides into the blood in the presence of insulin. The triglycerides further accumulate in muscle cells, causing those cells too to become further resistant to insulin. The more the muscle cells are resistant to insulin, the higher blood levels of glucose become. It is essentially an out of control feed-back mechanism between an impaired fat metabolism and an impaired carbohydrate metabolism. If not controlled, the situation will progressively degenerate.

The increase in the levels of fat in the blood is extremely dangerous for the health of the heart and blood vessels. Cardiovascular disease is therefore very common in patients with hypertension. Fat is the macronutrient that has been shown to cause and to aggravate the symptoms of hypertension. Saturated fats are particularly dangerous, with levels in processed meats sufficient to cause and aggravate hypertension. Dietary intervention for both weight loss and weight maintenance for hypertension should eliminate or overly minimize the consumption of saturated fats and related animal products that have been shown to cause or aggravate hypertension. Note that there are some plant sources of high saturated fat, e.g. palm oil. In high stakes dieting such as is the case in hypertension, there should be no room for generalizations. Each food should be analyzed for its pertinent characteristics. This is exactly what the plateau-proof diet has done. Each food has been analyzed using simple math formulas that reflect the state-of-the-art in biomedical and clinical research. There is enough variability even among closely related foods, and generalizations will undoubtedly result in inefficiency in weight loss.

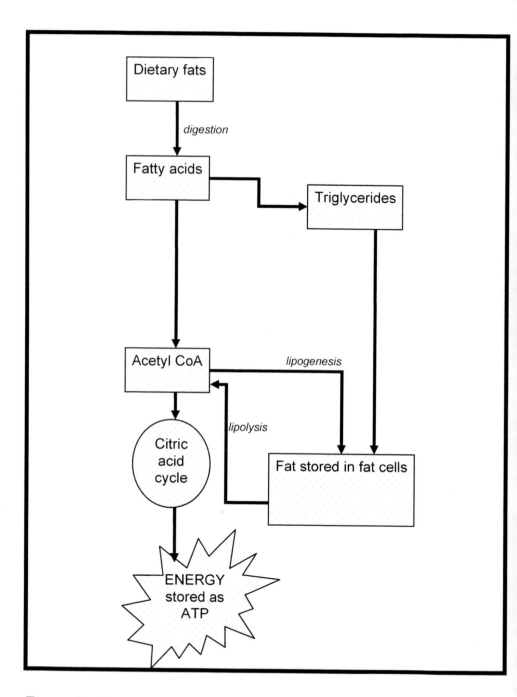

Figure 2 – Summary of fat metabolism.

Protein metabolism

Proteins are digested into amino acids in the stomach and intestines. These amino acids cross into the bloodstream through the small blood vessels that line the walls of the intestines. Several things can happen to these amino acids once they get into the bloodstream:

1) They may be used to synthesize proteins that are incorporated into the body (tissue protein). Our bodies are composed mostly of protein, and dietary protein is required for growth and maintenance.
2) They may be broken down into urea and excreted through the kidneys in urine.
3) Like glucose and fatty acids, they may be broken down into acetyl CoA and eventually to carbon dioxide and water. This process yields energy.
4) Under certain circumstances, amino acids may be converted to glucose (gluconeogenesis), or may be converted into fatty acids and stored in fat cells.

A summary of protein metabolism is shown in Figure 3.

It will be shown later that protein is the most important macronutrient for obesity and weight loss. In hypertension and obesity, the metabolism of both fat and carbohydrates is compromised. The metabolism of protein is normal during obesity, and numerous studies have shown that protein metabolism is normal in hypertension. Recent findings from medical research show that dietary protein has crucial roles to play in the course of weight loss (shown in later chapters). The plateau-proof diet takes advantage of these and other scientific facts to form the basis of the best weight loss diet ever known.

Protein and hypertension

The metabolism of protein appears to be normal or only slightly compromised in hypertension[110-122]. Some hypertension diets have cautioned against increasing the amounts of dietary protein for 2 reasons:

1) They are concerned that dietary protein may accelerate the course of kidney disease. Kidney disease is linked to hypertension and is likely to present sooner or later depending on the control of hyperglycemia.

2) They are concerned that deficiencies in protein metabolism resulting from hypertension may lead to toxicity.

It is true that high protein diets may accelerate the course of kidney failure in uncontrolled hypertension, especially when it is aggravated by type II diabetes. When the hypertension and diabetes are under control, increasing the amount of protein in the diet has been shown to be a safe and efficient strategy in weight loss diet therapy[115,117,119,123-126]. As a matter of fact, dietary protein is inversely proportional to blood pressure[123].

Since type II diabetes occurs in most cases of idiopathic hypertension, diet therapy for type II diabetes is generally applicable to hypertension. A lot of diabetes diets do not distinguish between type I (insulin-dependent) and type II (insulin-independent) diabetes; an error of great magnitude. Although there are similarities between type I and type II diabetes, their differences are significant and warrant separate strategies for dietary intervention. In the case of protein metabolism for instance, while protein metabolism appears to be normal in type II diabetes, it is abnormal in type I diabetes. The deficiencies in protein metabolism that some healthcare professionals are concerned about, are characteristic of type I, but not type II diabetes.

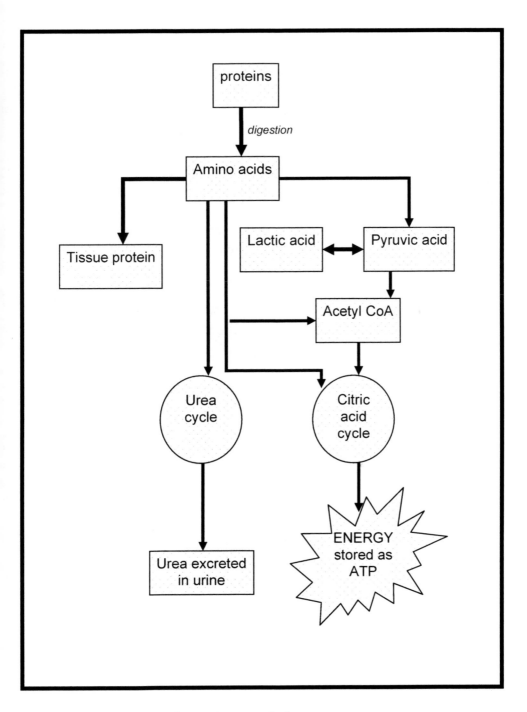

Figure 3 – Summary of protein metabolism.

Metabolism summary and discussion

The previous discussions on metabolism have accounted for the fate of dietary carbohydrates, fats and protein. There is constant breaking down and building up of glucose, fatty acids and amino acids in the cells of the body. The rate of breaking down to building up is an important factor in the dietary basis of obesity and the progression of hypertension and its associated diseases. In later chapters, it will be shown that the body can be adequately manipulated to burn more energy than it stores fat – which is the core of a successful and sustainable weight loss diet. As is shown in Figure 4, carbohydrates, fats and proteins can be converted, each to the others. This fact exposes a basis of the long-term failure of diets that favor excessive amounts of a particular nutrient while limiting another. There is usually a great deal of redundancy in the physiological processes in the body, and the body eventually adapts to almost any external or internal fluctuations from the norm. Diets such as the low-carb diets for example, affect an initial weight loss and the weight loss reaches a plateau, at which point further weight loss is impossible. The plateau is the point where weight loss stops prematurely, although the dieter is on the same diet. This is usually followed by a relapse into weight gain. This plateau phenomenon is not unique to low-carb diets. Low-fat diets and all other low calorie diets are limited by the plateau. As a matter of fact, there is no weight loss diet available today, other than the plateau-proof diet, that is not limited by the plateau. The plateau is the most frustrating element of weight loss dieting. The plateau-proof diet is aptly designed to eliminate the weight loss plateau; and it is unique and vastly distinguished in this capacity.

■

It is important to note that we have discussed metabolism in general, but specifics are a matter of individual variation. No two people are identical, and no two people have the exact body composition. Metabolic rates and the specifics of energy balance vary among individuals. If the human body was a combustion engine, it would generate 4 calories of energy for each gram of carb and protein, and 9 calories for each gram of fat eaten. It wouldn't matter if it was my body or yours. The human body is however not a combustion engine, and it doesn't follow the calorie-counting math. What a gram of carb does in my body is different from what a gram of carb does in your body. What happens to that gram of carb or fat is dependent on many factors that we as scientists are only now beginning to understand. As a matter of fact, weight loss diets that are based on counting calories are obsolete, considering the state of knowledge from research in obesity and weight loss.

The fact that a calorie is not standard within a human and among humans makes counting calories for weight loss a futile exercise. A proper approach is to understand and apply the parameters that influence caloric variation to the core of the diet. This is exactly one of the things that the plateau-proof diet has accomplished.

■

Metabolism and body composition are dynamic, and therefore a successful weight loss diet must also be dynamic if it is going to be sustainable. One-dimensional weight loss diets that are based solely on the restriction of one macronutrient, e.g. the low-carb diets and the low-fat diets are static diets. These diets lack the dynamic capacity that is required to adapt to the changes in metabolism and body composition. The obvious fact is that the body adapts to these diets sooner or later. When this happens, weight loss from these diets reaches the plateau. The plateau-proof diet has addressed this problem by providing the first multidimensional and the first dynamic weight loss diet. Essentially, the plateau-proof diet is the only weight loss diet that can be used for long-term weight loss. Since obesity is a chronic problem, a weight loss diet can only be considered to be a treatment for obesity if it can work in the long-term. By this standard, the plateau-proof diet is the only weight loss diet that is a treatment for obesity.

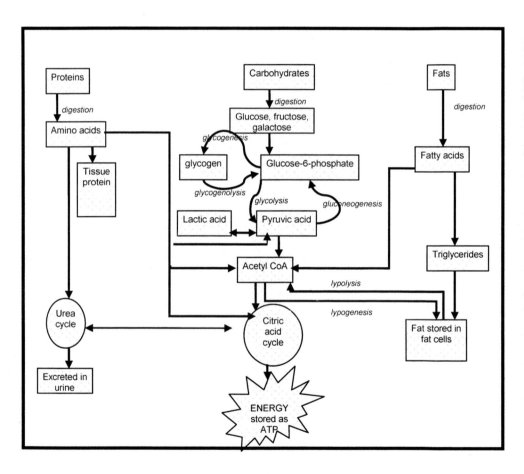

Figure 4 – Summary of carbohydrate, fat and protein metabolism.

Summary of metabolism in hypertension

Excessive body weight and obesity appear to be the most significant risk factors for hypertension. Amongst obese people, those with a greater proportion of visceral (gut) fat are at a higher risk of developing hypertension and its associated diseases. Visceral fat cells secrete fat more easily than subcutaneous fat cells. Aggravated by factors such as high fat, and the presence of certain animal products in the diet, visceral fat cells may increase their secretion of fat into the blood stream. The increased fat in the blood stream is absorbed into muscle cells where it is used for energy under normal circumstances. When the level of fat in the blood is persistently high; however, some of the fat accumulates in muscle cells.

When fat accumulates in muscle cells, these cells lose their sensitivity to insulin. In other words, these cells become resistant to insulin. Under normal circumstances, insulin facilitates the entry and oxidation of both glucose and fat in these cells. As the cells become increasingly resistant to glucose, entry and oxidation of glucose and fat are increasingly impaired. The levels of glucose in the blood become higher than normal and the levels of fat in the blood also stay elevated.

Unlike carbs and fat, the metabolism of protein is either normal or only slightly compromised in hypertension. It is logical then to have protein at the core of any dietary intervention in hypertension. It will be shown later that protein deserves this role for many important reasons.

It is clear that excess body weight and fat are at the center of initiating and aggravating the symptoms of hypertension. Luckily, the symptoms of hypertension and some its related diseases are reversible with weight loss. The goal of this dietary intervention is to produce and maintain a weight loss that is accompanied by a decrease in the levels of fat and glucose in the blood. It is this type of weight loss that will reverse the symptoms of hypertension and the type II diabetes with which it is so often associated.

Chapter Two

The Fundamentals of Obesity and Weight loss

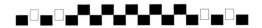

The aim of this chapter is to briefly discuss the fundamentals of obesity and the principles of weight loss dieting. The information in this chapter is particularly important for the following reasons:

1) Weight loss dieting is likely to be more effective in people who understand the source of their obesity. It is important that you take a minute to identify the cause of your obesity prior to starting the plateau-proof diet – you will get better results. The idea is simple; it is only after understanding the cause of your obesity that you are going to be able to make the lifestyle changes that may be necessary to facilitate your weight loss and the maintenance of your new trim look. Take for instance that the cause of your obesity is binge eating – obesity treatment will only work for you if you make a lifestyle change that addresses the overeating.

2) Knowing how to measure obesity and to recognize the types of obesity will offer you more control in your recovery. It is important to know your body in terms of where you are most likely to deposit fat, and where fat is shed the fastest while you are on the plateau-proof diet. You will see later that the plateau-proof diet is controllable, as is the rate of weight loss for dieters on the plateau-proof diet. It is ultimately up to the dieter to

accelerate or slow down the rate of weight loss. It is necessary to have a basic knowledge of obesity measurement for proper control of your weight loss.

3) Knowing the basic principles of weight loss dieting is beneficial for completely understanding how the plateau-proof diet works. Also in knowing the state of weight loss dieting today, it will be easy to appreciate why the plateau-proof diet is by a vast margin the best weight loss diet ever known to mankind.

Obesity

The word obesity originated from the Latin *obesus* (fat). Obesity is an increase in body weight to beyond normal, due to the excess accumulation of fat in the body.

What causes obesity?

<u>Genetics.</u> There is overwhelming evidence that obesity may be passed on from parents to kids. Just because everyone in your family is obese doesn't necessarily mean that you acquired obesity by heredity. People in the same family may have the same lifestyle or similar behaviors that cause obesity. There is no cause for alarm if obesity runs in your family – you should still be able to shed off the excess fat and maintain a fresh trim look with the plateau-proof diet.

Lifestyle and behaviors. Some of the most common causes of obesity are factors such as; what a person eats, how often they eat, eating due to boredom, eating for pleasure (even when not hungry), level of activity, etc. Identify which of these bad behaviors live(s) in your house and send it packing – you will experience great results with the plateau-proof diet.

Psychological factors. Some people react to negative emotions such as sadness, anger, feeling of inadequacy, etc. by overeating. Others react to all emotions by overeating. Some deal with stress by overeating. Some health professionals call this behavior *binge eating disorder*. If you suspect that you may be suffering from this disorder, please see a therapist prior to starting the plateau-proof diet. If you are unable or unwilling to see a therapist, do your best to recognize, acknowledge and address the problem.

Illnesses. There are certain illnesses that may cause obesity. These illnesses include hypothyroidism, Cushing's syndrome, depression, and other neurological disorders that result in overeating. In most people with obesity induced by illness, the plateau-proof diet will be effective for attaining and maintaining weight loss.

Drugs. Certain prescription drugs such as steroids and some antidepressants can cause obesity. Only a tiny fraction of obesity is from this etiology. If the drug is replaceable, that should be done. If the drug is not replaceable, weight loss is still possible (although relatively more difficult) with the plateau-proof diet.

Are there any health risks associated with obesity?

Obesity is not just about looking big. There are many health risks associated with obesity. A moderately obese person is at least twice as likely as a non-obese person to die prematurely. The risk of premature death increases linearly with weight, or degree and type of obesity. Obesity has been linked to heart disease, stroke, diabetes, high blood pressure, gout, sleep apnea (and other breathing disorders), osteoarthritis, gall bladder disease, gall stones, emotional disorders, colon cancer, rectal cancer, prostate cancer, ovarian cancer, cervical cancer, uterine cancer, breast cancer, cancer of the gall bladder, etc. Apple-shaped obese people are at a higher risk for heart disease, hypertension, and cancer than pear-shaped people of equal weight.

■

How is obesity measured?

There are many methods available for measuring obesity. It is however sufficient for most people to simply stand on a weight scale. You need to know just one thing when it comes to obesity measurement – the ideal weight range for your height. This number is an important number because it forms the core of your weight loss goal(s) on the plateau-proof diet, and lets you know when to start the weight maintenance diet. There is a chart in Appendix I that has height to weight indices.

The most accurate method for measuring obesity involves weighing a person under water. This method is complicated and requires the use of sophisticated equipment. It is unnecessary to go through the trouble. Other less accurate methods include measuring skin fold thickness in many areas of the body, and bioelectric impedance analysis – a technique in which small electrical currents are sent through the body.

I wouldn't recommend these methods as they are both high in error rate.

A good way to measure obesity uses the weight-for-height tables or the body mass index (BMI) table. This method is fast, simple, reliable, and doesn't require any special equipment. Basically, you match up your weight and height on a chart (like that in Appendix I) to determine if you are normal, overweight, or obese.

■

The waist-to-hip ratio

The waist-to-hip ratio is used to determine if a person is apple-shaped or pear-shaped. Most disease risk factors are greater in apple-shaped obesity than in pear-shaped obesity. The plateau-proof diet is capable of rapidly and preferentially reducing gut fat, thereby reducing the risk of disease in apple-shaped obesity. To get the waist-to-hip ratio, measure the waist at the narrowest point (x) and measure the hips at the widest point (y). Divide (x) by (y) [x/y] – this is the waist-to-hip ratio. If you are a woman with a ratio greater than 0.8, you are apple-shaped. If you are a man with a ratio greater than 1.0, you are apple-shaped.

Obesity and hypertension

Obesity is a leading cause of hypertension. It was shown in the previous chapter how excess fat can cause and aggravate hypertension and its associated diseases. Fortunately, the symptoms of hypertension can be reversed with weight loss[119,124,127-132]. Weight loss in hypertension is more challenging compared to weight loss in normal health. The main challenges are:

1) The efficacy of weight loss diets is lower in people with hypertension than in normotensive obese or overweight individuals. It is not surprising that weight loss diets do not work well for individuals with hypertension. These weight loss diets were not designed for hypertensive patients. In hypertension, there are significant changes in the way the body functions. These changes are many and are significantly far away from the norm to warrant a special weight loss diet. Up until now, the popular weight loss diets have not addressed the case of hypertension. Other diets address metabolic factors such as control of hyperglycemia, but they do not exploit the peculiarities of hypertensive metabolism for efficient weight loss. The plateau-proof diet for hypertension is designed to be an efficient weight loss diet. It has taken advantage of the peculiarities of metabolism in hypertension to correct the inadequacies that make conventional and popular weight loss diets less efficient for patients with hypertension.

2) Safety for hypertensive patients is not addressed by most of the conventional and popular weight loss diets. The deficiencies in fat and carbohydrate metabolism that are characteristic of hypertension must be controlled by dietary intervention. There are many different versions of and recommendations for hypertension diets. These diets are typically not designed for weight loss, for which reason they are of limited beneficial

impact to the majority of the cases of hypertension. Type II diabetes is very commonly associated with hypertension, and hypertensive patients often are advised to follow diabetic diet regimens. Most of these diets make no distinction between type I and type II diabetes. Type I and type II diabetes are significantly different in important factors, and each merits a distinct dietary approach. These diets are also too general to be of significant therapeutic value to most hypertensive individuals. Some of these diets, for example, may consider groups of foods such as fruits and vegetables as good, and other groups as bad. These recommendations are just too general to be effective. In developing the plateau-proof diet, it was obvious that foods need to be analyzed individually rather than clustered in groups. With the plateau-proof diet, one vegetable may be listed in a 'green' table and another in a 'red' table. The defining characteristics of both the disease and the individual foods have to be considered in developing a safe and efficient weight loss and/or weight maintenance diet for hypertension.

Confused by the many diets and dieting terminology?

Well, not after you read this. This section describes all the types of weight loss diets worth talking about, and breaks down the jargon.

Types of weight loss diets

1) *Hypocaloric diets.* These are weight loss diets that restrict the amount of calories allowed per day (low calorie diets). The rationale behind these diets is to consume less energy than the amount of energy required by the body. In a rather simplistic way, it appears logical that the balance of the energy is going to come from energy stores (fat) in the body. These diets typically affect an initial weight loss in most people. The weight loss eventually hits a plateau, after which people tend to relapse into weight gain[133,134].

2) *The low-carb and very low-carb diets.* These are low calorie diets in which the energy restriction is due to a decrease in the amount of carbohydrates in the diets. The popular low-carb diets typically substitute the carbs for fat. There is no consensus as to what amount of carbs distinguishes the low-carb diets from the very low-carb diets. It is common to refer to both simply as low-carb diets. These diets are effective for short-term weight loss, but the weight loss reaches a plateau relatively quicker than with other diets[129,135-144]. Since these diets allow for unrestricted amounts of saturated fats, they are potentially dangerous for cardiovascular health. These diets are incapable of attaining and maintaining complete weight loss for most people, and may be of limited use in the treatment of obesity. It is actually possible that most people on these diets will end up with the same amount of weight as they were when they started, and in addition develop cardiovascular disease from the high saturated fats in these diets.

3) *Low-fat diets.* The low-fat diets are also hypocaloric diets in which the energy restriction is from decreasing the amount of fat. Low-fat diets affect weight loss at a slower rate than the

low-carb diets; however, the weight loss reaches a plateau slower than with the low-carb diets[115,129,138,145-153].

4) *Ketogenic diets.* The ketogenic diets are very low calorie diets that cause an increase in the level of ketones in the blood (ketosis)[152-155]. The ketones come from the metabolism of fat, since these diets are typically high in fat and low in carbs. The ketones also come from the fat that is stored in the body. It was shown in the previous chapter that fat can be used for energy by all parts of the body except the brain and red blood cells. Ketosis makes the blood more acidic (reduce the pH of blood). Ketosis is essentially a state of blood toxicity (poisoning). It is believed that sustained ketosis may cause metabolic disorders as well as problems with the liver and kidneys. Some proponents of low-carb diets believe that the increase in blood ketones causes suppression of appetite; however, results from medical studies do not agree with that claim[135].

5) *High-fiber diets.* These diets reduce the amount of glucose absorbed into the blood stream by increasing the amount of indigestible carbs (fiber). Since human are incapable of digesting fiber, the fiber contributes to the bulk of the diet but not to its energy value. High-fiber diets can contribute to a limited extent in the treatment of obesity[156-169]. Diets rich in fiber have been shown to be beneficial for the health, including the facilitation of bowel movements and a reduction in the risk of certain cancers[170-187]. High-fiber diets are therefore a healthy way of lowering carbs. The plateau-proof diet uses a fiber index to incorporate foods that are rich in fiber.

6) *The protein-sparing diets.* Also called the protein-sparing modified fast, these diets typically allow only meats, fish and vegetables[188-204]. These are very low-carb hypocaloric diets that require close medical monitoring as they can cause severe

ketosis and cardiac arrhythmia (a type of heart failure)[205]. Initial weight loss is typically rapid, but these diets are obviously unsustainable.

Why is the plateau-proof diet superior to all of these weight loss diets?

The plateau-proof diet is vastly superior to existing weight loss diets because of two important factors.

(1) Weight loss dieting is simply a matter of manipulation of 3 macronutrients – carbs, fat and protein. It is clear from the previous section that all the weight loss diets either lower the amount of one macronutrient, e.g. low-carb, or they reduce the amount of total calories consumed. In other words, all the diets use a one-dimensional approach. Obesity is however a complex multidimensional problem and a one-dimensional approach is simply insufficient to treat it. The plateau-proof diet uses simple mathematical formulas that take into account all three of the macronutrients, based on their peculiar characteristics as determined by medical research. There is no macronutrient that is unaccounted for in the plateau-proof diet formulas. It will be shown later how this multidimensional approach to obesity treatment was developed. The plateau-proof diet attacks obesity from all the pertinent angles, providing the first treatment for obesity with this multidimensional capability.

(2) A common characteristic of all the existing weight loss diets is the weight loss plateau. This is the point where weight loss

stops prematurely although the diet and dietary habits are the same. The plateau-proof diet has innovatively addressed this problem by using a rotation system. The rotation system prevents the body from adapting to the diet, hence eliminating the weight loss plateau. Because of the rotation system, the plateau-proof diet is dynamic, whereas other existing weight loss diets are static. The human body is a dynamic entity that invariably adapts to things that cause changes to its norm. A low-carb diet, for example, is a deviation from what the body knows as normal. When the body is placed on the low-carb diet, it will invariably adapt to it, and the diet will no longer be able to cause weight loss. To prevent adaptation, the plateau-proof diet uses a simple rotation, making it the first dynamic weight loss diet.

It is mainly in being multidimensional and dynamic that the plateau-proof diet is vastly superior to all the existing weight loss diets; considering the fact that all existing weight loss diets are one-dimensional and static. There are other important ways in which the plateau-proof diet is superior to existing weight loss diets, for example; ease of use, controllability, sustainability, etc. All of these are going to be obvious to you when you start using the diet.

Popular Weight Loss Diets – where we were before the Plateau-proof Diet

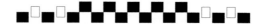

This chapter takes a deep look into the types of diets that have been proven to be effective for short-term weight loss in clinical trials. Close attention was paid to both the good and bad qualities of these diets in developing the plateau-proof diet. The plateau-proof diet improved on the strengths of these diets, and also made strength out of their weaknesses.

The results of dieting and weight loss from a large number of independent clinical trials were analyzed. A few of the representative results are summarized in this chapter. The summaries are followed by a lay interpretation and discussion of the clinical studies. It is important to look at a large number of independent dieting and weight loss clinical trials for the following reasons:

1) To demonstrate that the sample size (number of participants) across the multiple trials is large enough for the results to be statistically significant.

2) To demonstrate that the diet type and weight loss results are applicable to more than one population of people.

3) To accommodate for variations in degree of obesity of the participants in the various studies.

4) To accommodate for population lifestyle and behavioral differences among participants, and to understand the significance of these differences in relation to diet type and obesity.

5) Most importantly, to give the reader a realistic picture of the current state of dieting and weight loss, with an emphasis on the void that the plateau-proof diet has now filled.

The results of diet type and weight loss from the clinical trials discussed in this chapter are from industrialized nations across the world. The following types of diets and their weight loss results are discussed in this chapter:
- Low-carbohydrate and very low-carbohydrate diets
- High-protein diets
- Low-fat diets
- High-fiber diets
- Hypocaloric (low calorie) diets

There are obviously a number of diets that are neither worthy of clinical studies nor of your consideration; hence, are not mentioned in this book.

Low-carbohydrate, very low-carbohydrate, and low-fat diets

Low-carb diets are popular nowadays, with many Fad dieters using different variations of it. Low-carb diets have actually been around since the 1800s, and have been used therapeutically for the management of obesity. William Banting, for example, described his low-carb diet in the 1860s[206]. Banting, who was 66 years old at the time claimed to have benefited from appetite suppression from the diet, and a resultant weight loss of 46 pounds (initial weight was 202 lbs) in a one year period. He praised the diet for having an immediate effect; noticeable within a week.

We are a long way from Banting's days; however, the efficacy (effectiveness) and safety of low-carb diets are still a matter of debate and controversy. Proponents of the low-carb diets claim that these diets are relatively more effective for weight loss. Others claim that these diets can be used to cure obesity (as in get thin and stay thin). Opponents of the low-carb diets dispute the long-term efficacy and safety of these diets. They claim that these diets are likely to cause abnormalities in metabolism, which will lead to liver and kidney disease.

This section looks at the results of weight loss from low-carb and low-fat diets, and sheds light on their efficacy and safety. For simplicity, the clinical studies are summarized in tables. Each table is followed by a discussion of the study.

■■

Low-carb diet table 1.

Location / year of study	Virginia Polytechnic Institute, Blacksburg, VA USA. 2005
Diet type	Very low-carb (20 g per day for 2 weeks followed by an increase of 5 g per week for 10 weeks.
Average weight loss	8.3% of initial body weight – 7 Kg (15.4 lbs)
Duration of study	12 weeks
Number of participants	13
Special considerations	Study monitored blood and urine ketone levels. Ketone levels increased in week 1, then dropped progressively.

This trial[135] studied the effects of a very low-carbohydrate diet on 13 premenopausal women between the ages of 32 and 45. The study was done in an out-patient setting. The average initial weight of the participants was 84.8 Kg (186.9 lbs). Average weight loss at 12 weeks was 7 Kg (15.4 lbs). Prior to the start of the low-carb diet, the average energy from food for these women was 2,025 Kcal per day (49% carbs, 15% protein, 36% fats). Energy consumption at week 1 was 1,290 cal per day (10% carbs, 32% proteins, 57% fats), and at week 12 was 1,535 cal per day (15% carbs, 24% proteins, 61% fats).

The results of this study show a short-term decrease in body weight resulting from a low-carb diet. The duration of the study was too short to determine if further weight loss could be attained. Equally the duration of the study was not long enough to determine if the weight loss could be maintained, or if there was relapse into weight gain. The study did not address any safety parameters, but also did not report any immediate health complications from the participants. The sample size (number of participants in the study) is too small for the study to stand on its own.

Low-carb diet table 2.

Location / year of study	*University of Witwatersrand, Johannesburg, South Africa. 2000.*
Diet type	*Low-carb – 1600 Kcal (40% carbs, 30% proteins, 30% fats). Refined carbs were replaced with complex carbs. Saturated fats were replaced with unsaturated fats.*
Average weight loss	*7.7 Kg (17 lbs)*
Duration of study	*16 weeks*
Number of participants	*13*
Special considerations	*All participants were gout patients.*

This trial[141] studied the effects of a low-carbohydrate diet on 13 men between the ages of 38 and 62. The average weight of the participants at the beginning of the study was 91.1Kg (200.8 lbs), and average weight at 16 weeks was 83.4 Kg (183.7 lbs). Average weight loss at 16 weeks was 7.7 Kg (17 lbs). Participants decreased their dietary carbs, replacing them with proteins. Daily protein consumption was around 120 g. Dairy intake was limited as a source of protein, while poultry and fish were added in the diet to increase protein.

In addition to the weight loss, this low-carbohydrate diet also decreased fat and cholesterol levels in the blood. Blood levels of triglycerides (fat) dropped from 4.7mmol/l to 1.9 mmol/l. Blood levels of low density lipoprotein cholesterol (LDL-C), also known as bad cholesterol, dropped from 3.5 mmol/l to 2.7 mmol/l in 16 weeks. The results of this study suggest that short-term weight loss can be attained with a diet that is low in carbs. It goes further to show that a diet low in carbs and saturated fat, and high in protein may decrease risk factors (triglycerides and LDL-C) for heart disease.

The duration of the study is however too short to draw any inferences for the long-term. Also, the sample size (number of participants in the study) is too small for the study to stand on its own.

Low-carb vs low-fat diet table 3.

Location / year of study	Multicenter – headed in University of Pennsylvania School of Med. USA. 2003
Diet type	Very low-carb – 20 g / day in the first 2 weeks and gradual increase. No restriction in fats and proteins.
Average weight loss	9.6 Kg (21.2 lbs) after 6 months 7.2 Kg (15.9 lbs) after 12 months
Duration of study	12 months
Number of participants	63 (20 males & 43 females)
Special considerations	The study compared the efficacy of a low-carb diet to that of the conventional low-fat diet.

This study[136] involved two groups of participants – one on a very low-carb diet with no restrictions in fats and proteins, and the other on a conventional low-fat, hypocaloric (low calorie) diet. In the low-carb group, carb intake was limited to 20 g per day in the first 2 weeks of the study, and then slowly increased. The other group had a high-carb, low-fat diet with energy restrictions – 1200-1500 Kcal and 1500-1800 Kcal per day respectively for men and women. The diet was composed of about 60% carbs, 25% fats and 15% proteins. Age and obesity levels were similar in both groups.

The low-carb group lost weight faster than the conventional low-fat diet group – 21.2 lbs compared to 11.5 lbs at six months into the study.

This difference was smaller at 12 months into the study, with the low-carb group climbing to 15.9 lbs and the conventional diet group remaining almost unchanged at 9.7 lbs.

There was a significant decrease in the blood triglyceride (fat) levels in the low-carb group, which was sustained to the 12 month point. There wasn't a similar decrease in blood triglyceride levels in the conventional diet group. The conventional diet group; however, had a decrease in LDL-C (bad cholesterol) levels, which was not witnessed in the low-carb group. The lowering of both triglycerides and LDL-C in the low-carb group from *table 2*, was then likely due to the substitution of saturated fats with unsaturated fats and protein.

The dropout rate was high in this study, with only 59% of participants completing the study. The results of this study suggest that a low-carb diet may be more effective than a conventional low-fat diet for short-term weight loss. We see however that the low-carb diet reached a weight loss plateau after six months. After the plateau, there was relapse into weight gain (21.2 lbs lost after 6 months and 15.9 lbs lost after 12 months). The low-fat diet also hit a plateau by 12 months (11.5 lbs lost after 6 months and 9.7 lbs after 12 months).

Obesity is a chronic disease; therefore, dieting can only be an effective treatment for obesity if the diet is not limited by the weight loss plateau as is the case with the low-carb and low-fat diets. This is why the plateau-proof diet was developed – to conquer the weight loss plateau.

Low-carb vs low-fat diet table 4.

Location / year of study	University of Illinois at Urbana-Champaign. USA. 2003
Diet type	Low-carb low-fat – 1700 Kcal/day (30% proteins, 41% carbs, 29% fats)
Average weight loss	7.5 Kg (16.5 lbs)
Duration of study	10 weeks
Number of participants	24
Special considerations	This study compared a low-fat, low-carb diet to a low-fat, high-carb diet. 12 participants in each group.

The participants in this study[142] were 24 females ages 45 to 65. The study compared the effects of a low-carb diet to those of a low-fat, high-carb diet over a 10 week period. The low-carb diet consisted of 30% proteins, 41% carbs, and 29% fats, while the higher carb diet consisted of 16% proteins, 58% carbs, and 26% fat. Average weight loss in the low-carb group was 7.5 Kg (16. 5 lbs), compared to 6.96 Kg (15.3 lbs) in the higher carb group. The ratio of fat to lean tissue (muscle) loss was higher in the low-carb group.

The results of this study suggest that low-carb diets cause a more rapid short-term weight loss than low-fat diets. These results cannot be extrapolated to the long-term, since the trial time was too short. It however compliments other studies which have shown that low-carb diets are more effective than low-fat diets for short-term weight loss.

Low-carb diet table 5.

Location / year of study	Multicenter – Glasgow and Aberdeen, UK. 1996
Diet type	Low-carb – 1200 Kcal (35% of energy from carbs).
Average weight loss	5.6 Kg (12.3 lbs) at 3 months 6.8 Kg (14.9 lbs) at 6 months
Duration of study	6 months
Number of participants	110
Special considerations	Study compared low-carb and high-carb diet for weight loss and cardiovascular risk factors.

This study[143] involved 110 women ages 18 to 68. The women were divided into 2 groups; one group was placed on a low-carb diet and the other on a high-carb diet. Both diets provided the same amount of calories (1200 Kcal per day). In the low-carb diet, carbs contributed 35% of the calories, while in the high-carb diet; carbs contributed 58% of the calories. At 3 months the high-carb group lost an average of 4.3 Kg (9.5 lbs) and the low-carb group lost an average of 5.6 Kg (12.3 lbs). In the high-carb group, total cholesterol level in the blood was lowered as were levels of LDL-C (bad cholesterol). In the low-carb group total triglycerides (fat) were lowered, but there was no improvement in blood cholesterol levels.

At 6 months the high-carb group lost an average of 5.6 Kg (12.3 lbs), and the low-carb group lost an average of 6.8 Kg (14.9 lbs). Blood cholesterol levels remained lower in the high-carb group, and blood triglyceride levels were lowered too. In the low-carb group, blood triglyceride levels stayed lower, however there was no improvement in total blood cholesterol levels, and other risk factors for cardiovascular disease.

The results from this study indicate that short-term weight loss can be attained using either a high-carb or low-carb diet. These results also suggest that there is another factor (other than the lowering of carbs) that affects weight loss. We are going to see later that this factor is protein.

Weight loss with the low-carb diet was more rapid than weight loss with the high-carb diet, which is consistent with the results of the previously discussed studies. The risk factors for cardiovascular disease were improved on the high-carb diet, but not on the low-carb diet. We are beginning to see that low-carb diets with unrestricted fat intake may pose a threat to cardiovascular health.

Low-carb vs low-fat diet table 6.

Location / year of study	University of Guelph, Ontario, Canada. 2004
Diet type	Very low-carb – very low energy (766.8 Kcal/day) - 15.4% of energy intake from carbs.
Average weight loss	7.0 Kg (15.4 lbs)
Duration of study	10 weeks
Number of participants	31
Special considerations	This study compared a very low-carb and low-fat diet for weight loss and cardiovascular disease risk factors.

This study[129] involved 31 men and women 24 to 61 years old. The 10 week study compared the effect of a very low-carb and a low-fat diet on weight loss and blood levels of cardiovascular disease risk factors. Total energy from food was extremely low in both diets – 766.8 Kcal per day for the very low-carb diet, and 609.6 Kcal per day for the low-fat diet. At 10 weeks the very low-carb group lost an average of 7.0 Kg (15.4 lbs) and the low-fat group lost an average of 6.8 Kg (14.9 lbs). This study, like the others, supports the observation that low-carb diets and very low-carb diets provide a faster rate of weight loss than low-fat diets. It is important to note that the previous studies compared diets that provided the same daily amounts of calories (isocaloric diets). In this study the low-fat diet had fewer calories than the low-carb diet; however, weight loss was greater in the low-carb group than in the low-fat group. This shows that weight loss is not just a matter of calories, and the management of weight loss should not be limited to caloric restriction.

The other results of this study showed an improvement in cardiovascular risk factors in the low-fat group, but not in the low-carb group. Total cholesterol and LDL-C (bad cholesterol) were lowered in the low-fat group at 10 weeks. This is consistent with the findings in the previous studies, supporting the observation that low-fat diets are superior to low-carb diets in lowering the risk factors of cardiovascular disease.

Low-carb vs low-fat diet table 7.

Location / year of study	*Sakura Hospital, School of Medicine, Japan. 2003*
Diet type	*Low-carb (1000 Kcal / day total energy with 25% proteins, 40% carbs, and 35% fats).*
Average weight loss	*9.0 Kg (19.8 lbs)*
Duration of study	*4 weeks*
Number of participants	*22*
Special considerations	*This study compared a low-carb diet and a low-fat diet for weight loss and visceral (gut) fat in obese diabetes patients.*

The participants in this study[144] were 22 obese diabetes patients. They were divided into 2 groups, and placed on either a low-carb diet or a low-fat diet. Both diets provided an equal amount (1000 Kcal) of daily energy (isocaloric). The low-carb diet consisted of 25% protein, 40% carbs and 35% fats. The low-fat diet consisted of 25% protein, 65% carbs, and 10% fats. At 4 weeks, the low-carb group lost an average of 9.0 Kg (19.8 lbs) and the low-fat group lost an average of 7.0 Kg (15.4 lbs). The quantity of visceral (gut) fat was also measured. The low-carb group lost 4 times more visceral fat than the low-fat group.

The results of this study are consistent with those of previous studies which show that low-carb diets are superior to low-fat diets for attaining short-term weight loss. Like some of the other studies we have discussed, the duration of this study (4 weeks) was too short to extrapolate the long-term effects, in terms of efficacy and safety, of low-carb diets on weight loss management.

This study however suggests an important characteristic of low-carb–induced weight loss. It shows that there may be more targeting and reduction of visceral fat with low-carb diets than with low-fat diets. Other studies have supported this finding. The significance of this is that a more rapid reduction of visceral fat will more quickly lower the risk of some obesity-related diseases. Previous studies showed that certain cardiovascular risk factors are reduced with low-fat diets, but not with low-carb diets. This and other studies suggest that low-carb diets may have their own selective ability in lowering disease risk by rapidly decreasing visceral fat. These are all important factors that we will consider later in the book, when discussing the scientific basis, efficacy, and safety of the plateau-proof diet.

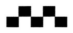

Low-carb vs low-fat diet table 8.

Location / year of study	Philadelphia VA medical center, USA. 2003
Diet type	Low-carb with total carbs limited to under 30 g per day.
Average weight loss	5.8 Kg (12.8 lbs)
Duration of study	6 months
Number of participants	132
Special considerations	This study compared the effects of a low-carb diet and a low-fat diet on weight loss.

This study[138] compared the weight loss efficiency of a low-carb versus a low-fat diet. There were 132 participants in this study. A significant number of the participants had either diabetes or metabolic syndrome. The minimum age of the participants was 18. The low-carb group had no restrictions on fat intake, but was instructed to limit carbs to 30 g per day or less. This group was also advised to consume fruits and vegetables with high-fiber content. The low-fat group had 30% or less of total daily calories from fat. At 6 months, the low-carb group lost an average of 5.8 Kg (12.8 lbs) and the low-fat group lost an average of 1.9 Kg (4.1 lbs).

The results of this study support those of the previous studies, in showing that low-carb diets are more efficient than low-fat diets for short-term weight loss.

Low-carb vs low-fat diet table 9.

Location / year of study	Multicenter – U. of Pennsylvania Health System, USA. 2004
Diet type	Low-carb – not more than 30 g per of carbs. Diet consisted of 25% proteins, 32% carbs, and 43% fats.
Average weight loss	8.5 Kg (18.7 lbs)
Duration of study	6 months
Number of participants	78
Special considerations	This study compared the weight loss efficiency of a low-carb diet and a low-fat diet.

78 participants completed this 6 month study[139]. The study compared the weight loss efficiency of a low-carb diet and a low-fat diet. 35 participants completed the low-fat program and 43 participants completed the low-carb program. Participants in the low-carb group

consumed no more than 30 g of carbs per day. The diet in the low-carb group consisted of 25% proteins, 32% carbs, and 43% fats. Participants in the low-fat group had around 30% or less of total daily calories from fats. Their diet consisted of 16% protein, 32% carbs and 43% fats.

At 6 months, the low-carb group lost an average of 8.5 Kg (18.7 lbs), and the low-fat group lost an average of 3.5 Kg (7.7 lbs). The study also measured levels of C-reactive protein (an indicator of inflammation) in the body. There was no significant difference between the 2 groups for levels of C-reactive protein. There was however a difference among the high risk (for inflammation) participants. Among the high risk participants, the low-carb diet showed a greater decrease in the levels of C-reactive protein than the low-fat diet. This indicates that a low-carb diet may be more efficient in reducing the risk of inflammation in high risk obese patients.

The results of this study support those of previous studies in showing that low-carb diets are more efficient than low-fat diets for short-term weight loss. The fact that low-carb diets may reduce inflammation, shows another benefit of low-carb diets that is lacking in conventional low-fat diets. Of course, we have to be mindful of the fact that low-carb diets with unrestricted fat pose a serious risk to cardiovascular health. We also have to be mindful of the fact that weight loss affected by low-carb diets is short-term, and it is equally likely that the reduction of inflammation risks may also be short-term. The weight loss plateau may not be the only plateau with these diets – also true for the other weight loss diets.

Low-carb vs low-fat diet table 10.

Location / year of study	Philadelphia VA medical center, USA. 2004
Diet type	Low-carb with total carbs limited to under 30 g per day.
Average weight loss	5.1 Kg (11.2 lbs)
Duration of study	12 months
Number of participants	132
Special considerations	This study compared the effects of a low-carb diet and a low-fat diet on weight loss.

This study[140] was a follow-up study from the study in *Low-carb diet table 8*. The study compared the efficiency of a low-carb diet versus a conventional low-fat diet for weight loss. The initial study was reported at 6 months from the start of the diet program. This study shows weight loss figures at 12 months. At 12 months, the low-carb group lost an average of 5.1 Kg (11.2 lbs), compared to 5.8 Kg (12.8 lbs) at 6 months. The low-fat group lost an average of 3.1 Kg (6.8 lbs) at 12 months, compared to 1.9 Kg (4.1 lbs) at 6 months. The results of this study show that although the low-carb diets have a rapid effect on weight loss, there are ineffective in causing additional weight loss in the longer term (plateau). The low-fat diets on the other hand, do not show a rapid effect on weight loss; however, their weight loss effect is sustained over a longer period of time. It takes longer for weight loss to plateau with low-fat diets compared to low-carb diets.

The results of these weight loss diets are representative of the trends in the population at large. The major frustration in weight loss dieting reported by most people is the weight loss plateau. Obesity is a chronic condition, and as such requires treatments that are effective in both the short-term and long-term. All of the current weight loss diets are ineffective for the treatment of obesity due to their limitation by the weight loss plateau. It is again for this reason that the plateau-proof diet was developed – to eliminate the weight loss plateau. Since it eliminates the weight loss plateau, the plateau-proof diet is the first and only dietary treatment for obesity.

Discussion on low-carb, very low-carb, and low-fat diets.

The low-carb and very low-carb diets are effective for short-term weight loss. Weight loss from these diets is more rapid than weight loss on low-fat diets, even when the diets are isocaloric (have the same amount of calories). Results from some clinical studies have also shown a greater amount of weight loss from low-carb diets, compared to low-fat diets, even when the low-carb diets had significantly more calories. These results indicate that a calorie from fat is not the same as a calorie from carbs. More appropriately, since we eat grams of fat and gram of carbs rather than calories of fat and calories of carbs – the relative caloric values of isocaloric (absolute) fat and carb are not equal. In other words, your weight loss diet is seriously flawed if it is based on counting calories. It will be shown later that a calorie from protein is also different from a calorie from fat and carbs.

The clinical research studies also show that weight loss reaches a plateau significantly faster with the low-carb diets than with the low-fat diets. This suggests that the body adapts to the low-carb diets a lot faster than it adapts to the low-fat diets. These findings suggest that the macronutrients themselves, and NOT the calories, affect their short-term and long-term fates in metabolism.

These findings, amongst others, have an influence in the invention and development of the novel weight loss diet and dieting techniques on which you are about to embark. Factors of most significance from these findings include:

1) The realization that diet programs that are based simply on counting calories are fundamentally flawed, and consequently limiting in their ability to affect a successful and sustainable weight loss.

2) The realization that very different molecular (very small) pathways are involved in the metabolism of carbohydrates, fats and proteins. The fact that it takes the body a significantly longer time to adapt to a low-fat diet, compared to a low-carb diet, indicates that the very small driving forces of metabolism are divergent (not influenced by the same factors in the body) for each of the macronutrients.

3) A successful and sustainable weight loss diet must be macronutrient driven, rather than calorie driven. The weight loss plateau is macronutrient-dependent; therefore, the plateau can be eliminated by macronutrient manipulation (as is the case with the plateau-proof diet).

These findings are not entirely surprising, considering what is already known about the metabolism of the macronutrients. For example, as was shown in chapter one, all carbohydrates are converted to glucose, which is the start point of carbohydrate metabolism. Fats on the other hand are converted into fatty acids. It was also shown in chapter one that not all parts of the body can use fatty acids for energy. The brain and the red blood cells do not use fatty acids for energy. When glucose is unavailable in the diet, the body is able to convert fatty acids into glucose, a nutrient that is used by all cells in the body for energy. The metabolic fate of dietary and stored fat is therefore determined by the relative amounts of fats and carbohydrates in the diet, in the first instance, rather than the amount of calories in the diet.

■

Some cohorts of low-carb dieters believe that the ketosis from very low-carb diets have an appetite suppressant effect. Ketosis is the presence of unusually high amounts of ketones (products of fat metabolism) in the blood. Glucose from carbs is the preferred source of energy in the body. In the absence of glucose in the diet, or in certain disease conditions such as diabetes, fat is converted into ketones and used for energy. Ketones make the blood acidic; hence ketosis is not a preferred state of the body. The body has mechanisms to automatically adjust the acid/base balance of blood. These mechanisms are called homeostasis. One aspect of homeostasis may be to restrict further breakdown of stored fat. This is likely one of the ways that the body adapts to low-carb diets.

There is no evidence that very low-carb ketogenic diets suppress the appetite. One study reported appetite suppression with a low-carb diet, but this appetite suppression lasted for only a month. Other studies have failed to establish a relationship between increased ketone levels in the blood and weight loss[135]. There is no scientific evidence to favor very low-carb ketogenic diets as opposed to relatively non-ketogenic low-carb diets. Ketogenic diets may not be a healthy long-term option for weight loss dieting, and they should be avoided.

■□■

Are low-carb diets safe?

Results from several clinical trials that compared low-carb diets to low-fat diets raise a serious concern about the safety of low-carb diets. In all the low-carb diet studies where fat was unrestricted, the level of LDL-C (bad cholesterol) in the blood was elevated, while blood levels of HDL-C (good cholesterol) was decreased or unchanged. The increase in the blood levels of bad cholesterol in low-carb diets presents a risk for cardiovascular disease. Low-carb diets that place no restriction on saturated fats are therefore dangerous to the health of the heart, and are likely to cause or aggravate the symptoms of hypertension. The low-carb diets however showed some beneficial effects on health, in addition to weight loss. Some studies showed that visceral (gut) fat is preferentially and more rapidly reduced with low-carb diets than with the conventional low-fat diets. Gut fat presents a greater risk of cardiovascular disease than subcutaneous fat (the fat under the skin). Low-carb diets have also been shown to reduce the chances of inflammation in obese people who are most at risk of it. In terms of safety therefore, low-carb diets are a little good and very bad.

The problem with the low-carb diets is that they are grossly one-dimensional. The issue of how the one-dimensional nature of these diets limits their efficiency is clearly seen in their inability to cause a sustainable weight loss. These low-carb diets, like other weight loss diets are useless for long-term weight loss – being limited by the weight loss plateau. It is the one-dimensional nature of these diets also that make them particularly dangerous for cardiovascular health as well as for aggravating the symptoms of hypertension. The weaknesses of the low-carb and low-fat diets were studied and used to strengthen the plateau-proof diet for hypertension.

Are low-carb and low-fat diets effective treatments for obesity?

In order to answer this question, we must look once more at the nature of obesity. Obesity is a chronic condition, which means it can be controlled with effective treatment, but it cannot be cured. Obesity cannot be cured because the things in the metabolism and the brain that cause obesity are dynamic (continuously in effect). For a diet to be able to control obesity in the long-term the diet must also be dynamic, else the body is going to adapt to it. When the body adapts to a diet, weight loss stops (the plateau), and even further restrictions of that diet are ineffective in causing more weight loss. This is the major problem with the efficiency of the low-carb and low-fat diets. The low-carb diets affect a relatively rapid initial weight loss, but they are limiting in that the body adapts to them rapidly. The low-fat diets don't affect weight loss as rapidly; however, they take a relatively longer time to plateau. The problem of the plateau is not limited to the low-carb and low-fat diets; all diets available today are equally limited. Almost all diets that are available today are capable of affecting an initial weight loss. The diets differ in the amount of the initial weight loss, but are all similar in being limited by the plateau. It was shown in the previous sections that the factors that affect metabolism of the macronutrients are multidimensional. The reality is that obesity is a chronic, dynamic, and multidimensional condition. The low-carb diets and other weight loss diets are static and one-dimensional. By what logic can anyone consider any of the weight loss diets available today as an effective long-term solution for obesity? Using any of these weight loss diets is comparable to betting on a sprinter in a marathon. It is exactly for this reason that the plateau-proof diet was developed. As will be shown later, it is the first and only dynamic and multidimensional diet – the minimum essential requirement for a weight loss diet to be invincible to the plateau.

High-protein or high-fat?

Proteins and fats are unrestricted in most low-carb diets, and it is up to the dieter to determine the ratio of these macronutrients in their diet. This one-dimensional approach to macronutrients is a major limiting factor of the low-carb and other weight loss diets. It is now obvious that 1 calorie from protein is different from 1 calorie from fat, and they are both different from a calorie from carb. It is not the absolute value of the calorie that is being considered; rather, it is the relative value of the calorie that is of interest. Basic laws of physics (thermodynamics) will argue that a calorie is a calorie regardless of its origin, and that 1 calorie from fat will do the same amount of work as 1 calorie from protein and 1 calorie from carb. A more profound fact however is that we don't eat calories – we eat grams of carbs, grams of fat, and grams of protein. It is what happens to these macronutrients when they get into the body that distinguishes their caloric contribution to the energy pool. The fate of each of the macronutrients is distinct, and is determined by the relative amount of the macronutrients rather than by calories.

There is an abundance of research data in favor of protein over fat as the replacement for reduced carbs in a low-carb diet[115,119,146,149,152,207-222]. Going by absolute caloric contribution, high-protein is the logical choice, considering that 1 g of fat contains more than twice the calories of 1 g of protein. There are other characteristics of high-protein diets that make them advantageous over high-fat diets. The other advantages of a high-protein to fat ratio include:

- The induction of thermogenesis (an energy consuming process during which the body produces heat). The increase in thermogenesis causes an increase in the expenditure of energy that would otherwise be stored as fat. Studies have shown that the rate of consumption of dietary energy is significantly higher when the diet is high in protein[212,215,220,221,223-227]. This phenomenon is called diet-induced thermogenesis (DIT). It is mainly due to proteins, as DIT from the other macronutrients is insignificant for weight loss. This energy is used to generate heat. It is a desirable thing to lose excess energy as heat, rather than store it as fat.

- More satiety (fullness) with a high-protein diet than with a high-fat diet. People tend to get full faster on a high-protein diet than on a high-fat diet[220,221]. This advantage of a high-protein diet cannot be overemphasized. A lot of obesity is caused by, or aggravated by overeating. A diet high in protein will help in solving the problem of overeating.

- A more favorable cardiovascular profile, in terms of lowering the risk factors of heart disease[115,119,149]. Whereas diets high in fat, particularly saturated fats, have been shown to increase the risk for heart disease; high-protein diets have been shown to have a favorable effect on the risk of heart disease.

- Proteins may increase the rate of burning stored fat. Studies have shown that high-protein in the diet have a direct effect on increasing the rate of breakdown of fat that is stored in fat cells[228,229].

- A high-protein diet is particularly effective in decreasing gut fat. This is another way in which a high-protein diet will contribute to a favorable cardiovascular profile. Additionally, it provides the esthetic value of a good waist to hip ratio.

- Long-term safety. High-protein diets are safe for long-term use[115,146,210].

- Increased protein in the diet may trigger the secretion of growth hormone during weight loss[230-233]. Growth hormone helps the body to stay lean, and its secretion is suppressed in obesity[234]. Growth hormone secretion may be regained with weight loss[230,235]. If growth hormone secretion is regained after weight loss, it is easier to maintain the new lean figure. If weight loss is not accompanied by the secretion of growth hormone, there is likely to be a relapse into weight gain. Not all weight loss diets trigger growth hormone secretion with weight loss[236].There is evidence that high-protein diets may be particularly favored in the secretion of growth hormone during weight loss.

- The last but certainly not the least advantage of a high-protein diet to a high-fat diet, is that protein metabolism in hypertension and obesity is normal. Fat metabolism on the other hand is severely compromised. In hypertension and obesity fat is the major part of the problem (most visible part anyway) – not the solution.

High-fiber and low glycemic load diets

High-fiber diets are basically less restricting low-carb diets. Fiber is a type of carbohydrate that is not absorbed into the bloodstream when it is eaten. Humans don't have the enzymes that are required to breakdown fiber into glucose; therefore fiber contributes to the bulk of food but not to the calories. Foods that are rich in fiber have a low energy density. Energy density is simply the amount of calories that are in one gram (or other unit) of carbohydrate. In the absolute sense, 1 gram of all carbohydrates has 4 calories of energy. One gram of a carbohydrate food that is made up of 50% fiber has an equal amount of calories (4) as 1 gram of sugar. The food that has 50% fiber will however provide only 2 calories of energy to the body, since half of it cannot be absorbed into the bloodstream. If you were trying to reduce the amount of carbs in your diet, for example, you could either eat half a gram of sugar or 1 gram of the food that has 50% fiber. In either case you will end up absorbing 2 calories worth of glucose into your bloodstream.

There is clinical and anecdotal evidence supporting a positive role of high-fiber diets in affecting weight loss[156-158,160,162-165,169,237]. These diets don't produce as rapid a weight loss as the very low-carb ketogenic diets. Weight loss with the high-fiber diets however doesn't plateau as rapidly as it does with the very low-carb ketogenic diets.

■

Low glycemic load diets are similar to high-fiber diets[238]. The low glycemic load diets also select carbohydrates with low energy densities. What distinguishes the low glycemic load diets from the high-fiber diets is that the low glycemic load diets emphasize the rate of absorption of glucose into the bloodstream. In other words, these diets favor high-fiber carbohydrates that are more slowly absorbed as glucose into the bloodstream. In terms of weight loss, the low glycemic load diets have no advantage over the high-fiber diets. Low glycemic load diets however, may have an advantage over regular high-fiber diets in obese patients with hypertension. Glucose metabolism is impaired in hypertension, making the blood glucose levels higher than normal. Since the low glycemic load diets release glucose into the bloodstream at a slower pace, they may help control the level of glucose in the blood after meals.

As will be shown later, the formulas for the plateau-proof diet take both amount of fiber and the equivalence of glycemic load into account.

The Plateau-proof Diet™ for Hypertension – Reversing the symptoms of hypertension with an efficient and sustainable weight loss

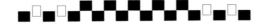

The science behind the plateau-proof diet

Having read the previous chapters, the following scientific facts on obesity and weight loss should now be almost obvious:

1) Weight loss is not merely a matter of thermodynamics. The old notion of counting the calories of the foods we eat is as obsolete as the science that created it. With the current state of knowledge from medical research, it is clear that weight loss diets that focus on counting calories (based solely on caloric restriction) are fundamentally flawed. A calorie from carbohydrates is different from a calorie from fats, and both are different from a calorie from protein. We saw clearly in the preceding chapter that an isocaloric (same number of calories) low-carb and low-fat diet consistently affect different degrees of weight loss. The low-carb weight loss diets consistently affected a more rapid weight loss than the low-fat diets. Weight

loss affected by the low-carb diets; however, reached a plateau faster than weight loss affected by the low-fat diets. The fact that isocaloric low-carb and low-fat diets have such distinct weight loss profiles reinforces the simple point that fat and carbs are metabolized in different pathways. It was shown in chapter one that these pathways can cross-talk (converge) with each other, however, it appears that the pathways tend to diverge more than they converge. Whatever the case may be, what is clear is that a calorie from carb is different from a calorie from fat and from a calorie from protein. Although in absolute terms, a gram of carbs equals 4 calories, and a gram of fat and protein equal 9 and 4 calories respectively, it is the relative caloric contribution to obesity or weight loss of each of these macronutrients when they enter the body that is of importance in obesity and weight loss. A gram of carb sitting in the refrigerator has 4 calories; does it generate 4 calories of energy when it gets into the body? What about the calories from a gram of fat or a gram of protein in the body? The relative caloric contribution of these nutrients is the energy balance in the body after the nutrients are eaten. It is deceptive to think that because you counted 500 calories for your lunch, your body is going to generate 500 calories of energy. We don't eat calories, we eat grams of food. The generation and expenditure of calories are different for each of the 3 macronutrients – carb, fat and protein. The fates of these macronutrients are determined by their relative abundance (ratio) in the diet, and not by the amount of calories in the diet.

2) The metabolism of fat and carbohydrate is severely compromised in hypertension. Protein metabolism on the other hand is either normal or only slightly compromised. A short-term increase in the amount of dietary protein is generally well tolerated, while short-term increases in fat and carb tend to

aggravate the symptoms of, and accelerate the progression of hypertension.

3) Proteins induce thermogenesis (the burning of calories as heat in the body) shortly after they are eaten. This phenomenon is referred to as diet-induced thermogenesis (DIT). Neither carbs nor fats display significant DIT for weight loss. Knowing this fact, no carbs or fats should enter the body unaccompanied by protein. Protein is the least compromised (in terms of metabolism) of the 3 macronutrients, and the only one that induces thermogenesis. It is exactly what is desired for weight loss – to burn energy rather than store it as fat. To reiterate, it is critical for weight loss to not let any fats or carbs into the body if these are unaccompanied by protein.

4) Diets that are rich in protein may induce the secretion of growth hormone during weight loss. Growth hormone secretion is compromised during obesity. Growth hormone is however essential for maintaining a trim look. When weight loss diets emphasize an increase in proteins, the secretion of growth hormone may be resumed faster with weight loss. It is easier to maintain the new trim look when growth hormone is helping. We now realize that not only are proteins vital for affecting weight loss; they may be equally vital for maintaining weight loss.

5) Weight loss diets that are rich in protein produce a more favorable cardiovascular profile than other diets. In particular, there is a remarkable improvement in blood pressure and blood triglyceride (fat) levels with weight loss. Protein-rich diets are quite a contrast from some of the more popular low-carb diets, which are essentially fertilizers for heart disease. Of course the best cardiovascular profile is achieved when saturated fats are decreased.

6) Proteins may increase the rate of burning of stored fat. Studies have shown that high-protein in the diet may have a direct effect on increasing the rate of breakdown of the fat that is stored in fat cells.

7) A high-protein weight loss diet is particularly effective in decreasing gut (visceral) fat. This is another way in which a high-protein diet will contribute to a favorable cardiovascular profile. Additionally, it provides the esthetic value of a good waist-to-hip ratio.

8) Protein rich diets affect satiety (feeling of fullness) faster than other diets, and therefore help to control over-eating.

9) Increased amounts of dietary protein have been shown to be safe for patients with hypertension and associated type II diabetes[115,117,119,125,210].

10) Doubling the amount of dietary protein neither affects renal function nor the progression of renal failure[115,117,119,125,210].

11) Proteins from plant sources, such as soy, lower the level of glucose in the blood[239,240].

12) Amino acids may regulate the secretion of insulin, and high protein diets improve plasma insulin responses[111].

13) There is an inverse relationship between blood pressure and dietary protein, and low-protein diets may aggravate hypertension[123,241-245].

14) Obesity is a dynamic and multidimensional problem; however, all the available weight loss diets are static and one-dimensional; hence, the weight loss plateau.

The logic behind the food tables – how The Plateau-proof Diet works, and why it is the best weight loss diet by a vast margin

The plateau-proof diet has captured all of the significant facts from medical research in hypertension, obesity, and weight loss and combined them into 2 simple mathematical equations. These equations have been used to assign indices (numbers) to more than a thousand foods – the lower the number the better the food for weight loss. These foods are found in the 'green', 'yellow' and 'red' tables below. The diet is the easiest weight loss diet to follow, as will be shown later in the simple instructions. Basically, all that is required is to choose foods in the 'green' tables to lose weight, while avoiding foods in the 'red' tables. To maintain the fresh trim look after weight loss, foods may be chosen from both the 'green' and 'yellow' tables. Isolated items in the 'yellow' tables may be chosen during the weight loss phase to make a balanced diet. The diet does not require the counting of calories, as this is already accounted for in the mathematical equations. The dieter has to eat less than 400 grams of food per day. Although less food will result in more rapid weight loss, food amounts should not be reduced to a point where sustainability is compromised.

■

The first of the 2 equations is called the CP (carb/protein) formula and the second is called the FP (fat/protein) formula. The CP formula takes the following into account: thermogenesis from protein, calories contributed by carb and protein, the fiber content of the carbs, the degree of refining of carbs, and the amount of saturated fats. The FP formula takes the following into account: thermogenesis from protein, the calories contributed by fat and protein, the degree of refining of carbs, and the amount of saturated fats.

Each formula has been used to make a distinct set of 'green', 'yellow' and 'red' food tables. There are 2 'green' tables to choose foods from, and 2 'red' tables to avoid. There are also 2 'yellow' tables to choose foods from during the maintenance stage of your weight loss, or to make a balanced diet during the weight loss stage.

There are two sets of tables for an important reason. If the body is placed on the same weight loss diet, it is going to adapt to that diet at some point, and weight loss is going to stop (the plateau). This is the main limitation of all the existing weight loss diets. To solve the plateau problem, the plateau-proof diet has used a multidimensional approach in including the multiple pertinent weight loss parameters in its formulas, and a dynamic approach in using a rotation system. The plateau-proof diet requires rotation of the CP and FP tables. As will be shown in the instructions, foods are chosen from the CP 'green' table for 4 weeks then from the FP 'green' table for 1 week. This rotation is necessary to prevent the body from adapting to the diet. It also makes the dieting less stressful by providing a broader selection of foods to choose from. This rotation also makes the plateau-proof diet the easiest diet to adhere to. Since it offers such a large number and broad variety of foods to choose from, the plateau-proof diet, as well as being the most effective, is also the least expensive to follow. It is simply a matter of comparing your grocery list with one 'green' (and 'yellow') list for 4 weeks and with another 'green' (and 'yellow') list for 1 week. The CP and FP formulas have done all of the work, and all that is required from the dieter is to choose foods from the 'green' and 'yellow' tables and avoid foods from the 'red' tables.

■

The CP and FP formulas

The CP and FP formulas in the most basic sense ensure that no carbs or fats enter the body unaccompanied by protein. This is the single most important thing to consider for a successful long-term weight loss. Why do we need protein to accompany the carbs and fat in the diet? As was shown previously, there are several reasons why protein should be the standard. These reasons are important and merit another look:

1) Protein triggers thermogenesis shortly after it is eaten. The body burns energy as heat during the process of thermogenesis. In the absence of thermogenesis, this energy would be stored as fat in the body. Since neither carbs nor fat induce thermogenesis, it is not such a bright idea to swallow them down without the right amount of protein.

2) The metabolism of fat and carbohydrate is severely compromised in hypertension. Protein metabolism on the other hand is either normal or only slightly compromised. A short-term increase in the amount of dietary protein is generally well tolerated, while short-term increases in fat and carb tend to aggravate the symptoms of, and accelerate the progression of hypertension.

3) Protein may trigger the secretion of growth hormone during weight loss. Growth hormone secretion is essential to maintain a lean body. In obesity the secretion of growth hormone is compromised, and the blood level of growth hormone drops. Weight loss by itself may not trigger the release of growth hormone; however, weight loss on a high-protein diet may

trigger release of growth hormone. It is easier to maintain weight loss when growth hormone is present in the blood.

4) Proteins may increase the rate of burning of stored fat. Studies have shown that high-protein in the diet have a direct effect on increasing the rate of breakdown of fat that is stored in fat cells.

5) A high-protein weight loss diet is particularly effective in decreasing gut (visceral) fat. This is another way in which a high-protein diet will contribute to a favorable cardiovascular profile. Additionally, it provides the esthetic value of a good waist-to-hip ratio.

6) Diets rich in protein affect satiety (feeling of fullness) faster, hence minimizing the risk of over-eating.

7) Increased amounts of dietary protein have been shown to be safe for patients with hypertension and the commonly associated type II diabetes.

8) Doubling the amount of dietary protein neither affects renal function nor the progression of renal failure.

9) Proteins from plant sources, such as soy, lower the level of glucose in the blood.

10) Amino acids may regulate the secretion of insulin, and high protein diets improve plasma insulin responses.

11) There is an inverse relationship between blood pressure and protein, and low-protein diets may aggravate hypertension.

12) Obesity is a dynamic and multidimensional problem; however, all the available weight loss diets are static and one-dimensional; hence, the weight loss plateau.

These are just some of the many reasons why protein is at the core of the plateau-proof diets, and why the CP and FP formulas tag dietary carbohydrate and fat to protein.

Derivation of the CP formula for hypertension

The first step in the derivation of the CP formula considers the number of calories provided by 1 gram of protein and 1 gram of carbs. It starts by multiplying the number of calories to number of grams.

Therefore;

For carbs (C) = 4 calories x 1g carb (since 1 gram of carbs gives 4 calories)

For proteins (P) = 4 calories x 1g protein (1 gram of protein also gives 4 calories)

The second step in the derivation of the CP formula considers thermogenesis. Proteins induce thermogenesis and are assigned a thermogenesis index of 2, while carbs are assigned a thermogenesis index of 1 since they don't induce thermogenesis. The thermogenesis index is then divided by the number of calories.

Therefore;

For carbs (C) = (4 calories x 1g carb) / 1

For protein (P) = (4 calories x 1g protein) / 2

The next step is to get the CP formula. To get the CP formula simply divide (C) and (P) from above.

Therefore;

CP = [(4 calories x *1g carb) / 1] / [(4 calories* x *1g protein) / 2]*

Which simply amounts to CP = 2 x *grams of carbs / grams of protein*
The formula is not yet complete since it hasn't accounted for the fiber content of the carbs. The next step of the formula multiplies the number of grams of carbs by the fiber index.

Therefore;

CP = (2 x grams of carbs x *fiber index*) / *grams of protein*

Below are the assigned indices for fiber:

- Very high-fiber = 0.25
- High-fiber = 0.50
- Moderate fiber = 0.75
- Low or no fiber = 1.00

The fiber index is important since it accounts for the difference in absolute caloric contribution from carbs that are absorbed into the bloodstream and those that are not (fiber).

The next step adds a saturated fat index to the formula:

$$CP = [(2 \text{ x grams of carbs x fiber index) / grams of protein}] + SFi$$

SFi is the saturated fat index.

Saturated fats have been shown to aggravate the symptoms, and to accelerate the co-morbidities of hypertension. Also, saturated fats in the diet are the main source of blood LDL-C, which accompanied with hypertension greatly increase the risks of cardiovascular disease. This is why the plateau-proof diet uses a saturated fat index. The index is designed to eliminate foods that contribute more than 20% of their total fat as saturated fat.

Derivation of the saturated fat index

The first step in the derivation of the saturated fat index divides total fat by unsaturated fat (total fat / unsaturated fat).

A hundredth of a point (0.01) is added to CP and FP for every hundredth (0.01) increase in (total fat / unsaturated fat) between 1 and 1.24. When (total fat / unsaturated fat) = 1.25, 20% of fats are saturated.

When (total fat / unsaturated fat) values are greater than or equal to 1.25, a tenth of a point (0.1) is added to CP and FP for every hundredth point (0.01) increase in the value of (total fat / unsaturated fat).

Further modification of the CP formula for hypertension

The formula above is good for weight loss in general, but it is further modified for increased safety and efficacy in hypertension. To create the most efficient weight loss diet for weight loss in hypertension, two additional indices are included in the formula;

1) **The perfect cardio index (PC*i*).** This index assigns numbers to animal food products that have been shown to induce, aggravate or accelerate the symptoms of hypertension and its co-morbidities. The goal is to limit or eliminate these foods from the diet. 10 points are assigned to all meats and meat-containing products, while 20 points are assigned to animal fat products and processed meats.

2) **The post-prandial (after meal) blood glucose index (PBG*i*).** This index distinguishes between highly refined, refined and unrefined carbs; favoring the consumption of unrefined carbs for controlling post-prandial blood glucose levels. The goal is to limit or eliminate carbs that rapidly increase the level of blood glucose. 5 points are assigned to highly refined carbs, 2.5 points to refined carbs, and 0 to unrefined carbs.

The final CP formula is therefore:

$$CP = [(2 \times grams\ of\ carbs \times fiber\ index) / grams\ of\ protein] + SFi$$

$$+ PCi + PBGi$$

What happens then to the formula when there is zero gram of protein or carb? 0 g is replaced with 0.0001g, since the formula assumes a seasoning effect. The seasoning effect is simply the fact that very small (trace) amounts of protein or carb may be derived from the seasoning(s) used in cooking, and therefore the absolute value of grams of carbohydrate or protein is never zero. Adjusting for the seasoning effect is insignificant and inconsequential to the output of the CP formula.

The lower the CP value, the better the food is for weight loss. Foods with the lowest CP values have been placed in the 'green' table ('Green' Rotation One Table), and are ideal for rapid weight loss. Foods with moderately higher CP values have been placed in the 'yellow' table ('Yellow' Rotation One Table), and are ideal for weight maintenance when used together with foods in the 'green' table. During the weight loss phase, isolated foods should be chosen from the 'yellow' tables to make a balanced diet with the foods in the 'green' tables. Foods in the 'red' table ('Red' Rotation One Table) must be avoided.

■

Derivation of the FP formula for hypertension

Like the CP formula, the first step in the derivation of the FP formula considers the number of calories provided by 1 gram of protein and 1 gram of fat. It starts by multiplying the number of calories to number of grams.

Therefore;

For fats (F) = 9 calories x 1g fat (since 1 gram of fat provides 9 calories)

For proteins (P) = 4 calories x 1g protein (1 gram of protein provides 4 calories)

The second step in the derivation of the FP formula considers thermogenesis. Proteins induce thermogenesis and are assigned a thermogenesis index of 2, while fats are assigned a thermogenesis index of 1 since they don't induce thermogenesis. The thermogenesis index is then divided by the number of calories.

Therefore;

For fats (F) = (9 calories x 1g fat) / 1

For protein (P) = (4 calories x 1g protein) / 2

The next step is to get the FP formula. To get the FP formula simply divide (F) and (P) from above.

Therefore;

FP = [(9 calories x 1g fat) / 1] / [(4 calories x 1g protein) / 2]

Which simply amounts to FP = 4.5 x grams of fat / grams of protein

Therefore;

FP = (4.5 x grams of fat) / grams of protein

The next steps add the saturated fat index, the perfect cardio index and the post-prandial blood glucose index. The final FP formula is therefore:

$$FP = [(4.5 \times grams\ of\ fat)\ /\ grams\ of\ protein] + SFi + PCi + PBGi$$

As was the case with the CP formula, the FP formula assumes the seasoning effect and replaces 0 g fat or 0 g protein with 0.0001g. Adjusting for the seasoning effect is insignificant and inconsequential to the output of the FP formula.

The lower the FP value, the better the food is for weight loss. Foods with the lowest FP values have been placed in the 'green' table ('Green' Rotation Two Table), and are ideal for rapid weight loss. Foods with moderately higher FP values have been placed in the 'yellow' table ('Yellow' Rotation Two Table), and are ideal for weight maintenance when used together with foods in the 'green' table. During the weight loss phase, isolated foods should be chosen from the 'yellow' tables to make a balanced diet with the foods in the 'green' tables. Foods in the 'red' table ('Red' Rotation Two Table) must be avoided.

How cutoff values of CP and FP were determined

The cutoff values of CP and FP are based on standardizing against the recommended diet of a healthy non-obese adult (25 year old) human. If all the recommended amounts of carbs, fats and proteins of a healthy non-obese adult were pooled together as one meal, the CP value for that meal will be approximately 12.0 and the FP value will be approximately 5.9.

The cutoff values of CP and FP for the plateau-proof diets are significantly below these values in the 'green' tables, and slightly below these values in the 'yellow' tables. Since obesity is a chronic condition, CP and FP values have to remain at these relatively low values even after complete weight loss has been attained. For this reason, it is highly recommended that during the maintenance phase (after desired weight loss has been achieved) foods should be chosen from both the 'green' and the 'yellow' tables, and never from the 'red' tables.

How to use The Plateau-proof Diet™

The plateau-proof diet for hypertension has 2 sets of tables – a CP set and an FP set. Each set consists of 3 tables; a 'green', a 'yellow' and a 'red'. The tables are listed in the pages below. The dieting essentially consists of eating foods listed in the 'green' tables for weight loss, and from the 'green' and 'yellow' tables for weight maintenance. Isolated food items should be chosen from the 'yellow' tables during the weight loss phase, in order to make a balanced diet with the food items in the 'green' tables. Food items in the 'red' tables are to be avoided. The dieting involves a rotation from the CP tables (4 weeks) to the FP tables (1 week), during the weight loss phase. If hypertension is reversed after weight loss, it is advisable to stay on the same rotation for weight maintenance. At this point more food may be chosen from the yellow tables as well as foods in the green tables. If weight loss does not reverse the hypertension; during the weight maintenance phase (after complete weight loss has been achieved) the rotations may be done in a 2 week equitemporal (equal amount of time) manner. That is, 2 weeks on the CP tables followed by 2 weeks on the FP tables. Close attention must be given to recording the body weight at this phase. If there is weight gain from changing to equitemporal rotations, then the rotations may be adjusted to spend more time in the CP tables. A 3 week (CP) to 1 week (FP) rotation, for example, may be ideal for some during the weight maintenance phase; and for others a 3 week (CP) to 2 week (FP) rotation may be ideal.

The first step in using the plateau-proof diet for hypertension is deciding how much weight to lose. Look up your ideal body weight in the chart in Appendix I. The chart shows the normal weight range for your height. Write down your target body weight in your weight loss log, and start following the diet as per the instructions below.

Record your weight into a log at the start of the diet. Record your weight on a weekly schedule for the entire duration of the diet. You may login to www.plataeuproofdiet.com to share your weight loss and weight maintenance progress with The Plateau-proof Diet Foundation. You could also subscribe to receive free copies of *Trimming America* (The Journal of The Plateau-proof Diet Foundation). This journal has updates and important tips on the plateau-proof diet as well as other important information on hypertension, obesity and weight loss.

How to use the plateau-proof diet

1) Start your diet with the CP (4 week) 'Green' Rotation One Table. Eat any items from this table for 4 weeks. Choose isolated items from the 'Yellow' Rotation One Table to make a balanced meal. Avoid all items in the 'Red' table. **Try to make a balanced meal out of the many items, and avoid eating the same items repeatedly.** [Note: if you are just getting off a

low-carb diet program, start the plateau-proof diet with FP (1 week) 'Green' Rotation Two Table].
*Eat a total of approximately 400 grams (14.1 ounces) or less of food per day – preferably spread out over 3 or more meals. (See Appendix II for sample 14 oz per day menu)

2) At the end of 4 weeks, eat any items from the FP (1week) 'Green' Rotation Two Table for 1 week. For most people the weight loss is going to be significantly less rapid than it was on the CP (4 week) 'Green' Rotation One Table. You must however complete this 1 week rotation before going back to the CP (4 week) 'Green' Rotation One Table. **Always try to balance your meals, and avoid eating the same items repeatedly.**

3) At the end of one week, go back to the CP (4 week) 'Green' Rotation One Table. Repeat steps (1) and (2) until you achieve your desired weight loss. When you achieve your desired weight loss, **choose foods equally from both the 'Green' and 'Yellow' tables to maintain your weight loss.** If your weight loss has reversed the hypertension, continue with the 4 week and 1 week rotations between the CP tables and the FP tables.

4) If your weight loss does not completely reverse your hypertension; during the weight maintenance phase (after complete weight loss has been achieved) the rotations may be done in a 2 week equitemporal (equal amount of time) manner. That is, 2 weeks on the CP tables followed by 2 weeks on the FP tables. Close attention must be given to recording the body weight at this phase. If there is weight gain from changing to equitemporal rotations, then the rotations may be adjusted to spend more time in the CP tables. A 3 week (CP) to 1 week (FP) rotation, for example, may be ideal for some during the

weight maintenance phase; and for others a 3 week (CP) to 2 week (FP) rotation may be ideal.

Weight loss profile of the plateau-proof diet

It must be pointed out here that we as humans are complex entities, and no two of us are alike. There is no treatment for any disease that works equally well for all patients. It is also true for the efficiency of weight loss with the plateau-proof diet, that there is going to be variation among the dieters. The diet is controllable, and that by itself empowers the dieter to control their rate of weight loss. For example, you are going to lose weight significantly faster on 250 g of food per day than on 400 g of food per day. Also, selecting foods with lower CP and FP values will result in a more rapid weight loss than foods with higher CP and FP values. Although selecting food items with lower CP and FP values in the 'green' tables will result in a more rapid weight loss than with higher CP and FP foods, it is strongly recommended that the emphasis be placed on having balanced meals. Remember that obesity treatment is a marathon, not a sprint – choose your foods to reflect this fact. A slower and sustainable weight loss on a balanced diet is ultimately healthier than a rapid unsustainable weight loss on a ketogenic diet.

So is there a predictable weight loss profile with the plateau-proof diet? Yes, there is. Most dieters will have 4 weeks of rapid weight loss followed by 1 week of slower (or no weight loss), then back to 4 weeks of relatively rapid weight loss, and so forth. The 4 week rotation 'green' tables (CP) are more efficient than the 1 week rotation 'green' tables (FP) for weight loss. The rotation is necessary to prevent the body from adapting to either diet; therefore, not only is it vital to follow the rotation, it is vital to select as broad a range of foods as possible within each table. When done properly, most dieters will have a relatively rapid weight loss with the CP rotations (4 weeks) and a slower weight loss with the FP rotations (1 week).

EAT FOODS FROM THIS TABLE FOR 4 WEEKS THEN SWITCH TO 'GREEN' TABLE TWO (DURING WEIGHT LOSS PHASE)

The Plateau-proof Diet 'Green' Rotation One Table (CP values)

ALFALFA SEEDS (SPROUTED, RAW)	1.5
ALMONDS (SLIVERED)	1.6
ANGLER	0.0
ASPARAGUS (CANNED)	3.0
ASPARAGUS (FROZEN)	1.5
BAMBOO SHOOTS (CANNED)	3.0
BASS	0.0
BEAN SPROUTS	2.5
BEET GREENS	3.0
BLACK BEANS (COOKED, DRAINED)	1.4
BLACK-EYED PEAS, DRY, COOKED	1.5
BLUE WHITING	0.0
BOUILLON (DEHYDRATED)	2.0
BRAZIL NUTS	1.5
BRILL	0.0
BROCCOLI (FROZEN, COOKED, DRAINED)	1.7
BROCCOLI (RAW, COOKED, DRAINED)	2.3
BRUSSELS SPROUTS	3.3
CABBAGE (CHINESE)	1.5
CARP	0.0
CASHEW NUTS (DRY ROASTD)	4.5
CASHEW NUTS (ROASTED, OIL)	3.5
CATFISH	0.0
CAULIFLOWER	4.5
CELERY (PASCAL, RAW)	2.0
CHICKPEAS	3.2
CHILI	2.4
CLAM CHOWDER (NEW ENGLAND, MILK)	3.8
CLAMS	0.4
CLUB SODA	2.0
COCKLE	0.0

COD	0.0
COFFEE	2.0
COLA (DIET)	2.0
COLLARDS	3.8
CONGER	0.0
CORN OIL	2.0
CRAB (BROWN MEAT)	0.0
CRAB (WHITE MEAT)	0.0
CRABMEAT	0.1
CUSTARD (BAKED)	4.5
DAB	0.0
DOGFISH	0.0
EEL	0.0
ENCHILADA (Vegetable or seafood)	2.4
ENDIVE	4.0
EVAPORATED MILK (NONFAT)	3.1
FILBERTS (HAZELNUTS)	2.4
FISH SANDWICH (NO CHEESE)	4.6
FISH STICKS	1.3
FLOUNDER	0.0
FLOUNDER (BAKED WITH VEGETABLE OIL)	0.0
FLOUNDER (BAKED, NO FAT)	0.0
GREAT NORTHERN BEANS (DRY, DRAINED)	2.9
GREEN PEAS (SOUP)	4.5
GREY MULLET	0.0
GURNARD	0.0
HADDOCK	0.0
HADDOCK (BREADED, FRIED VEGETABLE OIL)	0.8
HAKE	0.0
HAKE (S. AFRICAN)	0.0
HALIBUT	0.0
HALIBUT (BROILED, LEMON JUICE)	0.0
HERRING	0.0
HERRING (PICKLED)	0.0
JOHN DORY	0.0
KALE	3.5
KING CRAB (WHITE MEAT)	0.0
LEMON SOLE	0.0

LENTILS	1.2
LETTUCE (BUTTER-HEAD)	4.0
LETTUCE (CRISP-HEAD)	4.4
LETTUCE (LOOSE LEAF)	4.0
LIMA BEANS	3.1
LING	0.0
LIQUOR (GIN, RUM, VODKA, WHISKY, COGNAC...)	2.0
LOBSTER (BROWN MEAT)	0.0
LOBSTER (WHITE MEAT)	0.0
MACADAMIA NUTS (OIL ROASTED)	3.4
MACKEREL	0.0
MEGRIM	0.0
MILK (NONFAT)	2.7
MISO	4.6
MIXED NUTS (DRY ROASTED, NO HONEY)	2.6
MIXED NUTS (OIL ROASTED, NO HONEY)	1.8
MUSSEL	0.0
MUSTARD (YELLOW)	2.0
MUSTARD GREENS	2.0
NONFAT DRY MILK	3.0
NORWAY LOBSTER (WHITE MEAT)	0.0
NORWAY POUT	0.0
OCEAN PERCH (FRIED VEG OIL, BREADED)	0.9
OKRA	4.5
OLIVE OIL	2.0
OLIVES (BLACK)	2.0
OLIVES (GREEN)	2.0
ONIONS (RAW, SPRING)	4.0
OYSTER	0.0
OYSTERS (FRIED VEG OIL, BREADED)	2.0
OYSTERS (RAW)	0.8
PEA BEANS (DRY)	4.0
PEANUT BUTTER	1.2
PEANUT OIL	2.0
PEANUTS (VEG OIL-ROASTED)	1.3
PEAS (FRESH, GREEN)	4.3
PEAS (POD)	3.3
PECANS (HALVES)	5.0

PERCH	0.0
PILCHARD	0.0
PILCHARD (S. AFRICAN)	0.0
PINE NUTS	5.0
PINTO BEANS	4.9
PISTACHIO NUTS	1.8
PLAICE	0.0
POLLACK	0.0
PRAWN	0.0
PUMPKIN AND SQUASH KERNELS	1.4
RED KIDNEY BEANS	2.8
RED MULLET	0.0
REDFISH	0.0
REFRIED BEANS	4.3
RICOTTA CHEESE (NONFAT MILK)	0.9
SAFFLOWER OIL	2.0
SAITHE	0.0
SALMON	0.0
SALMON (CANNED)	0.0
SALMON (PACIFIC)	0.0
SALMON (RED, BAKED)	0.0
SALMON (SMOKED)	0.0
SAND EEL	0.0
SARDINES (CANNED, OIL, ATLANTIC)	0.0
SCALLOP	0.0
SCALLOPS (BREADED)	1.3
SEA BREAM	0.0
SEAWEED (SPIRULINA)	0.9
SESAME SEEDS	1.0
SHRIMP	0.0
SHRIMP	0.1
SHRIMP (FRIED, NOT BREADED, NOT BATTERED)	1.4
SKATE RAY	0.0
SNAP BEAN (GREEN)	4.5
SNAP BEAN (YELLOW)	4.5
SOLE	0.0
SOLE (BAKED, NO FAT)	0.0
SOY SAUCE	2.0

SOYBEAN OIL	2.0
SOYBEAN-COTTONSEED OIL	2.0
SOYBEANS	1.5
SPINACH (CANNED)	1.8
SPINACH (FRESH)	1.5
SPINACH (FROZEN)	2.5
SPRAT	0.0
SQUID	0.0
SUNFLOWER OIL	2.0
SUNFLOWER SEEDS	1.7
TACO	3.3
TAHINI	2.0
TEA (BREWED, UNSWEETENED)	2.0
TOFU	0.7
TROUT	0.0
TROUT (BROILED)	0.0
TUNA	0.0
TUNA (CANNED, LIGHT, OIL, DRAINNED)	0.0
TUNA (CANNED, LIGHT, WATER)	0.0
TURBOT	0.0
TURNIP GREENS (FROZEN)	3.2
TUSK	0.0
VINEGAR AND OIL SALAD DRESSING	2.0
WALNUTS (BLACK)	0.6
WALNUTS (ENGLISH)	1.9
WHITE SAUCE (NONFAT MILK)	4.2
YOGURT (NONFAT MILK)	2.8

EAT FOODS FROM THIS TABLE AND FROM 'GREEN' TABLE ONE FOR 4 WEEKS THEN SWITCH TO 'YELLOW' TABLE TWO (DURING WEIGHT MAINTENANCE PHASE). ALSO CHOOSE ISOLATED ITEMS FROM THIS TABLE TO MAKE A BALANCED DIET WITH ANY ITEMS IN 'GREEN' TABLE ONE.

The Plateau-proof Diet 'Yellow' Rotation One Table (CP values)

ALL-BRAN CEREAL	5.3
ARTICHOKES (GLOBE, COOKED)	6.0
AVOCADOS (CALIFORNIA)	6.0
BEEF (DRIED)	10.0
BEEF (LEAN, CHUCK BLADE)	10.0
BEEF (LEAN, BOTTOM ROUND)	10.0
BEEF BROTH (BOULLION)	10.0
BEEF HEART (BRAISED)	10.0
BEEF ROAST (LEAN, EYE O RND)	10.0
BEEF ROAST (LEAN, RIBS)	10.0
BEEF STEAK (LEAN, SIRLOIN, BROIL)	10.0
BEER (LIGHT)	10.0
CABBAGE (COMMON)	10.5
CABBAGE (RED)	6.0
CABBAGE (SAVOY)	6.0
CARROTS (FROZEN, COOKED)	9.0
CELERY SEED	10.0
CEREAL (100% NATURAL)	6.0
CHICKEN (CANNED)	10.0
CHICKEN (LIGHT & DARK, STEWED)	10.0
CHICKEN BREAST (FRIED VEG OIL, FLOUR)	10.1
CHICKEN BREAST (ROASTED)	10.0
CHICKEN DRUMSTICK (ROASTED)	10.0
CHICKEN DRUMSTICK, (FRIED VEG OIL, FLOUR)	10.2
CHICKEN LIVER	10.0
CHICKEN ROLL	10.2
CHOCOLATE (FOR BAKING, BITTER)	5.3
CHOW MEIN NOODLES	8.7

CLAM CHOWDER (MANHATTAN)	6.0
COCONUT (RAW)	10.5
CORN (RAW, WHITE)	9.5
CORNED BEEF (CANNED)	10.0
COTTAGE CHEESE (NONFAT)	10.5
CREAM OF MUSHROOM SOUP (WATER)	9.0
CUSTARD PIE	8.2
DANDELION GREENS	5.3
DUCK (ROASTED)	10.0
EGGS (FRIED VEG OIL)	10.3
EGGS (HARD-BOILED)	10.3
EGGS (POACHED)	10.3
EGGS (SCRAMBLED)	10.3
EGGS (WHITE, RAW)	10.0
EGGS (WHOLE, RAW)	10.3
EGGS (YOLK, RAW)	10.0
GROUND BEEF (BROILED, LEAN)	10.0
KOHLRABI	7.3
LAMB (LEG, LEAN, ROASTED)	10.0
LAMB CHOPS (ARM, LEAN, BRAISED)	10.0
LAMB CHOPS (LOIN, LEAN, BROIL)	10.0
LAMB RIB (LEAN, ROASTED)	10.0
LEMONS (RAW)	10.0
MELBA TOAST	8.0
MINESTRONE SOUP	5.5
MIXED GRAIN BREAD	9.4
MOZZARELLA CHESE (NONFAT MILK)	10.3
MUSHROOMS (CANNED)	5.3
MUSHROOMS (RAW)	6.0
OATMEAL (PLAIN)	9.0
ONION SOUP	8.0
PEAS (CANNED, GREEN)	5.3
PEPPERS (HOT GREEN CHILI)	8.0
PEPPERS (HOT RED CHILI)	8.0
PEPPERS (SWEET GREEN)	8.0
PEPPERS (SWEET RED)	8.0
POPCORN (AIR-POPPED)	9.0
POPCORN (VEGETABLE OIL)	9.0

PORK (LINK)	10.0
PORK (LUNCHEON MEAT, HAM, LEAN)	10.2
PORK (ROASTED HAM, LEAN)	10.0
PORK CHOP LOIN (BROILED, LEAN)	10.0
PORK CHOP LOIN (FRIED VEG OIL, LEAN)	10.0
PORK RIBS (ROASTED, LEAN)	10.0
PORK SHOULDER (BRAISED, LEAN)	10.0
RAISIN BRAN CEREAL	10.5
RYE BREAD (LIGHT)	8.6
SAUERKRAUT	7.5
SOLE (BAKED IN MARGARINE)	10.0
SPAGHETTI (FIRM)	8.4
SPECIAL K CEREAL	7.0
SQUASH (SUMMER)	8.0
STEAK (BROILED, SIRLOIN)	10.0
TOMATO JUICE	10.0
TOMATO SOUP (NONFAT MILK)	7.3
TOMATOES (CANNED)	10.0
TOMATOES (FRESH)	7.5
TORTILLAS (CORN)	9.8
TURKEY (LIGHT & DARK, ROASTED)	10.0
TURKEY (ROASTED)	10.0
TURKEY LOAF	10.0
TURNIP GREENS (FRESH)	6.0
VEAL CUTLET (BROILED, ROASTED, BRAISED)	10.0
VEAL RIB (BROILED, ROASTED, BRAISED)	10.0
VEGETABLE JUICE	8.3
VEGETABLES (MIXED)	5.6
VEGETARIAN SOUP	9.0
WAFFLES	7.7
WHEAT BREAD	10.1
WHEAT CRACKERS	10.0
WHIPPED TOPPING	7.0
WHOLE-WHEAT BREAD	7.2
WHOLE-WHEAT FLOUR	8.0
WHOLE-WHEAT WAFERS	7.5

AVOID THE FOODS IN THIS TABLE DURING THIS ROTATION

The Plateau-proof Diet '<u>Red</u>' Rotation One Table (CP values)

AMERICAN CHEESE	20.0
AMERICAN CHEESE SPREAD	20.8
ANGELFOOD CAKE	18.0
APPLE JUICE (CANNED)	58000.0
APPLE PIE	34.3
APPLE PIE (FRIED)	31.0
APPLES (RAW, UNPEELED)	480.0
APPLES (DRIED, SULFURED)	630.0
APPLESAUCE (CANNED, SWEETENED)	1020.0
APPLESAUCE (CANNED,UNSWEETENED)	560.0
APRICOT (CANNED, HEAVY SYRUP)	110.0
APRICOT NECTAR	72.0
APRICOTS (CANNED, IN JUICE)	31.0
APRICOTS (DRIED)	27.5
APRICOTS (RAW)	18.0
AVOCADOS (FLORIDA)	10.8
BAGELS (EGG)	10.9
BAGELS (PLAIN)	10.9
BANANAS	54.0
BARBECUE SAUCE	4000.0
BARLEY (PEARLED, LIGHT)	14.8
BEAN WITH BACON SOUP	12.9
BEANS (CANNED, FRANKFURTER)	11.7
BEANS (PORK, SWEET SAUCE)	13.4
BEANS (PORK, TOMATO SAUCE)	13.0
BEEF AND VEGETABLE STEW	11.4
BEEF GRAVY	12.4
BEEF LIVER (FRIED)	10.6
BEEF NOODLE SOUP	13.6
BEEF POTPIE	13.7
BEER (REGULAR)	26.0
BEETS (CANNED)	12.0

BEETS (COOKED, DRAINED)	14.0
BISCUIT BAKING MIX	14.0
BLACKBERRIES (RAW)	27.0
BLUE CHEESE	20.3
BLUE CHEESE SALAD DRESSING	22.0
BLUEBERRIES (FROZEN, SWEETENED)	100.0
BLUEBERRIES (RAW)	40.0
BLUEBERRY MUFFINS	13.3
BLUEBERRY PIE	28.7
BOLOGNA	20.6
BOSTON BROWN BREAD	21.0
BRAN FLAKES (40%)	11.0
BRAN MUFFINS	12.0
BRAUNSCHWEIGER	20.5
BREAD STUFFING (DRY MIX)	11.1
BREADCRUMBS	11.2
BROWN GRAVY (DRY MIX)	19.3
BROWNIES WITH NUTS	22.0
BUCKWHEAT FLOUR (LIGHT, SIFTED)	19.5
BULGUR	13.6
BUTTER	20.0
BUTTERMILK (DRIED)	22.9
BUTTERMILK (LIQUID)	23.4
CAKE & PASTRY FLOUR	21.7
CAMEMBERT CHEESE	20.0
CANDY (MILK CHOCOLATE, ALMONDS)	30.0
CANDY (MILK CHOCOLATE, PEANUTS)	26.5
CANDY (MILK CHOCOLATE, PLAIN)	36.0
CANDY (MILK CHOCOLATE, RICE CRISPIES)	38.0
CANTALOUP	22.0
CAP'N CRUNCH CEREAL	46.0
CARAMEL	44.0
CAROB FLOUR	42.0
CARROT CAKE (CREME CHESE FROSTING)	34.6
CARROTS (RAW)	12.0
CATSUP	27.6
CHEDDAR CHEESE	20.0
CHEESE CRACKERS (PEANUT SANDWICH)	20.0

CHEESE CRACKERS (PLAIN)	22.0
CHEESE SAUCE WITH MILK	22.9
CHEESEBURGER	23.7
CHEESECAKE	31.3
CHERRIES (RAW, SWEET)	22.0
CHERRIES (SOUR, CANNED, WATER)	44.0
CHERRY PIE	29.0
CHERRY PIE (FRIED)	32.0
CHESTNUTS (ROASTED)	30.4
CHICKEN A LA KING	10.9
CHICKEN AND NOODLES	12.4
CHICKEN BREAST (FRIED, BATTERED)	10.7
CHICKEN CHOW MEIN	15.1
CHICKEN DRUMSTICK (FRIED, BATTERED)	10.8
CHICKEN FRANKFURTER	21.0
CHICKEN GRAVY (CANNED)	15.2
CHICKEN GRAVY (DRY MIX)	19.3
CHICKEN NOODLE SOUP	14.5
CHICKEN POTPIE	13.8
CHICKEN RICE SOUP	13.5
CHOCOLATE (SWEET, DARK)	52.0
CHOCOLATE CHIP COOKIES	28.0
CHOCOLATE MILK (LOWFAT 1%)	16.5
CHOCOLATE MILK (LOWFAT 2%)	26.5
CHOCOLATE MILK (REGULAR)	26.5
CHOCOLATE PUDDING (nonfat milk)	13.5
CHOCOLATE SHAKE	35.0
CHOP SUEY (BEEF & PORK)	21.0
COCOA POWDER (NO FAT DRY MILK)	14.7
COCOA POWDER (REGULAR)	26.7
COCONUT (SHREDDED, DRIED, SWEETENED)	22.0
COFFEE CREAM (LIGHT)	13.0
COFFEECAKE (CRUMB)	16.7
COLA (REGULAR)	82000.0
CONDENSED MILK (SWEETENED)	33.8
CORN (CREAM, CANNED)	23.0
CORN (RAW, YELLOW)	14.3
CORN CHIPS	16.0

CORN FLAKES	24.0
CORN GRITS (WHITE)	20.7
CORN GRITS (YELLOW)	20.7
CORN MUFFINS	14.0
CORNMEAL	16.4
COTTAGE CHEESE (FRUIT)	22.9
COTTAGE CHEESE (LARGE CURDS, CREAMED)	20.4
COTTAGE CHEESE (UNCREAMED)	20.2
CRACKED-WHEAT BREAD	12.0
CRACKED-WHEAT BREAD	10.8
CRACKERS (SNACK)	40.0
CRANBERRY JUICE COCKTAL	76000.0
CRANBERRY SAUCE (SWEATENED, CANNED)	216.0
CREAM CHEESE	21.0
CREAM OF CHICKEN SOUP (MILK)	24.3
CREAM OF CHICKEN SOUP (WATER)	16.0
CREAM OF MUSHROM SOUP (MILK)	25.0
CREAM OF WHEAT	14.0
CREME PIE	35.1
CROISSANTS	10.8
CUCUMBER (WITH PEEL)	200.0
DANISH PASTRY (FRUIT)	14.0
DANISH PASTRY (PLAIN)	14.5
DATES	32.8
DEVIL'S FOOD CAKE (CHOCOLATE FROSTING)	28.7
DOUGHNUTS (CAKE TYPE, PLAIN)	16.0
DOUGHNUTS (YEAST-LEAVENED, GLAZED)	17.3
EGG NOG	17.6
EGG NOODLES	10.6
EGGPLANT	12.0
ENG MUFFIN (BACON, EGG, CHEESE)	23.4
ENGLISH MUFFINS (PLAIN)	10.8
EVAPORATED MILK (WHOLE)	22.9
FETA CHEESE	20.5
FIG BARS	31.5
FIGS (DRIED)	20.3
FISH SANDWICH (CHEESE)	24.9
FLOUNDER (BAKED IN BUTTER)	20.0

FRANKFURTER	20.4
FRENCH BREAD	10.7
FRENCH SALAD DRESSING (LOW CAL)	4000.0
FRENCH SALAD DRESSING (REGULAR)	2000.0
FRENCH TOAST	15.7
FROOT LOOPS CEREAL	25.0
FROSTED FLAKES CEREAL	52.0
FRUIT COCKTAIL (CANNED, HEAVY SYRUP)	96.0
FRUIT COCKTAIL (CANNED, JUICE)	58.0
FRUIT JELLIES	20000.0
FRUIT PUNCH DRINK (CANNED)	44000.0
FRUITCAKE	21.2
FUDGE, CHOCOLATE, PLAIN	42.0
GELATIN DESSERT	17.0
GINGER ALE	64000.0
GINGERBREAD CAKE	32.3
GOLDEN GRAHAMS CEREAL	24.0
GRAHAM CRACKER (PLAIN)	22.0
GRAPE DRINK (CANNED)	52000.0
GRAPE JUICE (CANNED)	76.0
GRAPE SODA	92000.0
GRAPEFRUIT (CANNED, SYRUP)	78.0
GRAPEFRUIT (RAW)	20.0
GRAPEFRUIT JUICE (SWEETENED)	56.0
GRAPEFRUIT JUICE (UNSWEETENED)	48.0
GRAPE-NUTS CEREAL	15.3
GRAPES (RAW)	1800.0
GROUND BEEF (BROILED, LEAN & FAT)	20.0
GUM DROPS	50000.0
HALF AND HALF (CREAM)	12.9
HAMBURGER	14.7
HARD CANDY	56000.0
HOLLANDAISE (WATER)	25.6
HONEY	558.0
HONEY NUT CHEERIOS CEREAL	15.3
HONEYDEW MELON	24.0
ICE CREAM (VANLLA,11% FAT)	33.4
ICE CREAM (VANLLA,16% FAT)	35.5

ICE MILK (VANILLA, 3%)	29.5
ICE MILK (VANILLA, 4% FAT)	31.3
IMITATION CREAMER (POWDERED)	2010.0
IMITATION SOUR DRESSING	22.8
IMITATION WHIPPED TOPING	2020.0
ITALIAN BREAD	12.8
ITALIAN SALAD DRESSING (LOW CAL)	400.0
ITALIAN SALAD DRESSING (REGULAR)	200.0
JAMS AND FRUIT PRESERVES	20000.0
JELLY BEANS	52000.0
JERUSALEM-ARTICHOKE	13.0
KIWIFRUIT	22.0
LAMB (LEG, LEAN & FAT, ROASTED)	20.0
LAMB CHOPS (ARM, LEAN & FAT, BRAISED)	20.0
LAMB CHOPS (LOIN, LEAN & FAT, BROIL)	20.0
LAMB RIB (LEAN & FAT, ROASTED)	20.0
LARD	2002.0
LEMON JUICE	32.0
LEMON MERINGUE PIE	20.5
LEMONADE	42000.0
LEMON-LIME SODA	78000.0
LUCKY CHARMS CEREAL	15.3
MACARONI	11.1
MACARONI AND CHEESE	24.7
MALTED MILK (CHOCOLATE)	26.4
MALTED MILK (REGULAR)	24.9
MALT-O-MEAL	23.0
MANGO (RAW)	70.0
MARGARINE (REGULAR, HARD)	12.0
MARGARINE (IMITATION 40% FAT)	12.0
MARGARINE (REGULAR, HARD, 80% FAT)	12.0
MARGARINE (REGULR, SOFT)	12.0
MARGARINE (REGULR, SOFT, 80% FAT)	12.0
MARGARINE (SPREAD, HARD, 60% FAT)	12.0
MARGARINE (SPREAD, SOFT, 60% FAT)	12.0
MARSHMALLOWS	46.0
MAYONNAISE (IMITATION)	4010.0
MAYONNAISE (REGULAR)	22.0

MAYONNAISE SALAD DRESSING	8020.0
MILK (1% LOW FAT)	13.0
MILK (2% LOW FAT)	22.7
MILK (WHOLE)	22.8
MOLASSES	44000.0
MOZZARELLA CHEESE (WHOLE MILK)	20.3
MUENSTER CHEESE	20.0
MUSHROOM GRAVY	18.7
NATURE VALLEY GRANOLA CEREAL	12.7
NECTARINES	32.0
OATMEAL & RAISIN COOKIES	24.0
OATMEAL (FLAVORED)	12.4
OATMEAL BREAD	11.2
ONION RINGS	16.0
ONIONS (RAW)	12.0
ORANGE & GRAPEFRUIT JUICE	50.0
ORANGE (RAW)	30.0
ORANGE JUICE (CANNED)	50.0
ORANGE JUICE (FRESH)	26.0
ORANGE SODA	92000.0
PANCAKES (BUCKWHEAT)	12.0
PANCAKES (PLAIN)	16.0
PAPAYA	34.0
PARMESAN CHEESE	20.2
PARMESAN CHEESE	20.2
PARSNIPS	22.5
PEACH PIE	30.1
PEACHES (CANNED, HEAVY SYRUP)	102.0
PEACHES (CANNED, JUICE)	29.0
PEACHES (DRIED)	32.7
PEACHES (FRESH)	20.0
PEANUT BUTTER COOKIE	14.0
PEAR (CANNED, HEAVY SYRUP)	98.0
PEAR (CANNED, JUICE)	64.0
PEAR (FRESH)	37.5
PECAN PIE	20.1
PICKLES (CUCUMBER)	600.0
PICKLES (CUCUMBER, DILL)	200.0

PICKLES (CUCUMBER, SWEET)	1000.0
PIE CRUST	14.1
PINEAPPLE (CANNED, HEAVY SYRUP)	104.0
PINEAPPLE (CANNED, JUICE)	78.0
PINEAPPLE (FRESH)	38.0
PINEAPPLE JUICE (UNSWEETENED)	68.0
PINEAPPLE-GRAPEFRUIT JUICE DRINK	46000.0
PITA BREAD	11.0
PIZZA (CHEESE)	25.6
PLANTAINS	42.8
PLUMS (CANNED, HEAVY SYRUP)	120.0
PLUMS (CANNED, JUICE)	76.0
PLUMS (FRESH)	18.0
POPCORN (SYRUP)	22.5
POPSICLE	36000.0
PORK (CURED, BACON)	20.0
PORK (CURED, CANADIAN BACON)	20.2
PORK (CURED, HAM, LEAN & FAT)	20.0
PORK (CURED, HAM, LEAN)	20.0
PORK (LUNCHEON MEAT, CANNED)	20.4
PORK (LUNCHEON MEAT, HAM, LEAN & FAT)	20.4
PORK CHOP LOIN (BROILED, LEAN & FAT)	20.0
PORK CHOP LOIN (FRIED, LEAN & FAT)	20.0
PORK FRESH (ROASTED HAM, LEAN & FAT)	20.0
PORK RIBS (ROASTED, LEAN & FAT)	20.0
PORK SHOULDER (BRAISED, LEAN & FAT)	20.0
POTATO CHIPS	20.0
POTATO SALAD (MAYONNAISE)	18.0
POTATOES (AU GRATIN)	32.4
POTATOES (BAKED, NO SKIN)	22.7
POTATOES (BAKED, WITH SKIN)	20.4
POTATOES (BOILED)	18.0
POTATOES (FRENCH FRIES, BAKED)	17.0
POTATOES (FRENCH FRIES, FRIED)	20.0
POTATOES (HASHED BROWN)	17.6
POTATOES (MASHED)	16.0
POTATOES (SCALLOPED)	32.4
POUND CAKE	19.8

PRETZELS	13.0
PRODUCT 19 CEREAL	16.0
PROVOLONE CHEESE	20.3
PRUNE JUICE	22.5
PRUNES (DRIED)	31.0
PUMPERNICKEL BREAD	10.6
PUMPKIN (CANNED)	13.3
PUMPKIN (FRESH)	12.0
PUMPKIN PIE	12.7
QUICHE LORRAINE	24.5
RADISHES	200.0
RAISIN BREAD	13.0
RAISINS	34.5
RASPBERRIES (SWEETENED)	55.5
RELISH (SWEET)	100.0
RHUBARB (SWEETENED)	150.0
RICE (BROWN)	20.0
RICE (WHITE)	25.0
RICE KRISPIES CEREAL	25.0
RICE PUDDING (nonfat milk)	13.5
RICOTTA CHEESE (WHOLE MILK)	20.5
ROAST BEEF SANDWICH	13.1
ROLLS (DINNER)	28.0
ROLLS (FRANKFURTER & HAMBURGER)	13.3
ROLLS (HARD)	12.0
ROLLS (HOAGIE OR SUBMARINE)	13.1
ROOT BEER	84000.0
RYE WAFERS (WHOLE-GRAIN)	15.0
SALAMI (DRY)	20.4
SALAMI (NOT DRY)	20.3
SALTINES	18.0
SANDWICH SPREAD (BEEF & PORK)	24.0
SAUSAGE (BROWN AND SERVE)	20.0
SEAWEED (KELP)	60.0
SELF-RISING FLOUR (UNSIFTED)	15.5
SEMI SWEET CHOCOLATE	37.7
SHEETCAKE (NO FROSTING)	26.3
SHEETCAKE (WHITE FROSTING)	51.3

SHERBET	55.2
SHORTBREAD COOKIE	20.0
SHREDDED WHEAT CEREAL	11.5
SNACK CAKES (DEVIL'S FOOD & CRÈME)	34.0
SNACK CAKES (SPONGE & CRÈME)	54.0
SOLE (BAKED IN BUTTER)	20.0
SOUR CREAM	22.9
SPAGHETTI (MEATBALLS, TOMATO SAUCE)	19.8
SPAGHETTI (SOFT)	12.8
SPAGHETTI (TOMATO SAUCE, CHEESE)	13.0
SPINACH SOUFFLE	20.5
SQUASH (WINTER)	18.0
STRAWBERRIES (FRESH)	15.0
STRAWBERRIES (FROZEN, SWEETENED)	55.5
SUGAR (BROWN)	424000.0
SUGAR (WHITE)	398000.0
SUGAR COOKIE	31.0
SUGAR SMACKS CEREAL	25.0
SUPER SUGAR CRISP CEREAL	26.0
SWEET POTATOE PIE	58000.0
SWEET POTATOES (BAKED)	21.0
SWEETPOTATOES (CANNED)	12.0
SWEETPOTATOES (CANNED, MASHED)	23.6
SWISS CHEESE	20.3
SWISS CHEESE	20.3
SYRUP (LIGHT, CHOCOLATE FLAVORED)	44.0
SYRUP (CORN, MAPLE)	64000.0
SYRUP (THICK, CHOCOLATE FLAVORED)	21.0
TANGERINE JUICE	60.0
TANGERINES (CANNED, LIGHT SYRUP)	82.0
TANGERINES (FRESH)	18.0
TAPIOCA PUDDING (nonfat milk)	18.7
TARTAR SAUCE	220.0
THOUSAND ISLAND DRESSING	420.0
TOASTER PASTRIES	38.0
TOMATO & VEGETABLE SOUP	12.0
TOMATO PASTE	10.9
TOMATO PUREE	12.5

TOMATO SOUP (WATER)	17.0
TOTAL CEREAL	14.7
TRIX CEREAL	25.0
TUNA SALAD (Imitation mayonnaise)	11.2
TURKEY AND GRAVY	12.0
TURKEY HAM (CURED)	20.0
TURKEY PATTIES (BATTERED, FRIED)	12.2
TURNIPS	16.0
VANILLA PUDDING (nonfat milk)	33.0
VANILLA SHAKE	29.1
VANILLA WAFERS	29.0
VEGETABLE & BEEF SOUP	12.5
VIENNA BREAD	13.0
VIENNA SAUSAGE	20.0
WATER CHESTNUTS	34.0
WATERMELON	23.3
WHEAT FLOUR (ALL-PURPOSE, SIFTED	14.7
WHEAT FLOUR (ALL-PURPOSE, UNSIFTED)	14.6
WHEATIES CEREAL	15.3
WHIPPING CREAM (HEAVY)	22.8
WHIPPING CREAM (LIGHT)	22.8
WHITE BREAD	12.0
WHITE BREAD CRUMBS	11.0
WHITE BREAD CUBES	15.0
WHITE CAKE (WHITE FROSTING)	31.2
YELLOW CAKE (CHOCOLATE FROSTING)	29.0
YOGURT (FRUIT, LOW FAT MILK)	28.6
YOGURT (PLAIN, LOW FAT MILK)	22.7
YOGURT (WHOLE MILK)	22.8

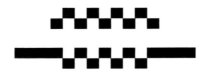

EAT FOODS FROM THIS TABLE FOR ONE WEEK THEN SWITCH TO 'GREEN' TABLE ONE (DURING WEIGHT LOSS PHASE)

The Plateau-proof Diet '<u>Green</u>' Rotation Two Table (FP values)

ALFALFA SEEDS (SPROUTED, RAW)	0.0
ALL-BRAN CEREAL	1.1
APPLES (DRIED, SULFURED)	0.0
APRICOTS (DRIED)	0.0
APRICOTS (RAW)	0.0
ARTICHOKES (GLOBE, COOKED)	0.0
ASPARAGUS (CANNED)	0.0
ASPARAGUS (FROZEN)	0.0
BARLEY (PEARLED, LIGHT)	0.6
BEAN SPROUTS	0.0
BEET GREENS	0.0
BEETS (CANNED)	0.0
BEETS (COOKED, DRAINED)	0.0
BLACK BEANS (COOKED, DRAINED)	0.3
BLACK-EYED PEAS, DRY, COOKED	0.4
BRAN FLAKES (40%)	0.0
BROCCOLI (FROZEN, COOKED, DRAINED)	0.0
BROCCOLI (RAW, COOKED, DRAINED)	0.0
BRUSSELS SPROUTS	0.8
BUCKWHEAT FLOUR (LIGHT, SIFTED)	0.8
BULGUR	0.8
CABBAGE (CHINESE)	0.0
CABBAGE (COMMON)	0.0
CABBAGE (RED)	0.0
CABBAGE (SAVOY)	0.0
CAROB FLOUR	0.0
CARROTS (FROZEN, COOKED)	0.0
CARROTS (RAW)	0.0
CAULIFLOWER	0.0
CELERY (PASCAL, RAW)	0.0
CHERRIES (SOUR, CANNED, WATER)	0.0

CHICKPEAS	1.3
CLAMS	0.4
COD	0.6
COLLARDS	0.0
CORN (CANNED)	1.1
CORN (RAW, WHITE)	1.5
CORN GRITS (WHITE)	0.0
CORN GRITS (YELLOW)	0.0
CRABMEAT	0.6
CRACKED-WHEAT BREAD	1.9
DAB	1.0
DATES	1.1
EGG NOODLES	1.3
EGGPLANT	0.0
EGGS (WHITE, RAW)	0.0
ENDIVE	0.0
EVAPORATED MILK (NONFAT)	0.2
FIGS (DRIED)	1.5
FLOUNDER	0.3
FLOUNDER (BAKED IN VEG OIL)	1.7
FLOUNDER (BAKED, NO FAT)	0.3
GRAPEFRUIT (RAW)	0.0
GREAT NORTHERN BEANS (DRY, DRAINED)	0.3
GREEN PEAS (SOUP)	1.7
GURNARD	1.8
HADDOCK	0.4
HAKE	0.8
HAKE (S. AFRICAN)	0.9
HONEYDEW MELON	0.0
JERUSALEM-ARTICHOKE	0.0
KALE	1.1
KING CRAB (WHITE MEAT)	0.2
KIWIFRUIT	0.0
KOHLRABI	0.0
LEMON SOLE	1.4
LEMONS (RAW)	0.0
LENTILS	0.3
LETTUCE (BUTTER-HEAD)	0.0

LETTUCE (CRISP-HEAD)	0.9
LETTUCE (LOOSE LEAF)	0.0
LIMA BEANS	0.3
MACARONI	0.6
MACKEREL	0.3
MILK (NONFAT)	0.5
MUSHROOMS (CANNED)	0.0
MUSHROOMS (RAW)	0.0
MUSTARD GREENS	0.0
NONFAT DRY MILK	0.1
NORWAY LOBSTER (WHITE MEAT)	0.3
OATMEAL (FLAVORED)	1.8
OKRA	0.0
ONION SOUP	0.0
ONIONS (RAW)	0.0
ONIONS (RAW, SPRING)	0.0
ORANGE (RAW)	0.0
OYSTERS (RAW)	1.0
PAPAYA	0.0
PARSNIPS	0.0
PEA BEANS (DRY)	0.3
PEACHES (DRIED)	0.8
PEACHES (FRESH)	0.0
PEAS (CANNED, GREEN)	0.6
PEAS (FRESH, GREEN)	0.1
PEAS (POD)	0.0
PEPPERS (HOT GREEN CHILI)	0.0
PEPPERS (HOT RED CHILI)	0.0
PEPPERS (SWEET GREEN)	0.0
PEPPERS (SWEET RED)	0.0
PILCHARD	0.9
PINTO BEANS	0.3
PLANTAINS (GREEN)	0.0
PLUMS (FRESH)	0.0
POTATOES (BAKED, NO SKIN)	0.0
POTATOES (BAKED, WITH SKIN)	0.0
POTATOES (BOILED)	0.0
PRAWN	1.4

PRUNES (DRIED)	0.0
PUMPKIN (CANNED)	1.5
PUMPKIN (FRESH)	0.0
RAISINS	0.9
RED KIDNEY BEANS	0.3
REDFISH	0.8
REFRIED BEANS	0.8
RICE (BROWN)	0.9
SALMON	0.5
SALMON (CANNED)	1.3
SALMON (RED, BAKED)	1.1
SAUERKRAUT	0.0
SCALLOP	0.9
SEAWEED (SPIRULINA)	0.6
SHRIMP	1.4
SHRIMP	0.2
SKATE RAY	1.7
SNAP BEAN (GREEN)	0.0
SNAP BEAN (YELLOW)	0.0
SOLE	1.0
SOLE (BAKED WITH VEG OIL)	1.7
SOLE (BAKED, NO FAT)	0.3
SOY SAUCE	0.0
SPAGHETTI (FIRM)	0.6
SPAGHETTI (SOFT)	0.9
SPINACH (CANNED)	0.8
SPINACH (FRESH)	0.0
SPINACH (FROZEN)	0.0
SQUID	1.4
SWEET POTATOES (BAKED)	0.0
SWEETPOTATOES (CANNED)	0.0
SWEETPOTATOES (CANNED, MASHED)	0.9
TANGERINES (FRESH)	0.0
TOMATO PASTE	1.0
TOMATOES (FRESH)	0.0
TUNA (CANNED, LIGHT, VEG OIL, DRAINNED)	1.4
TUNA (CANNED, LIGHT, WATER)	0.2
TURNIP GREENS (FRESH)	0.0

TURNIP GREENS (FROZEN)	0.9
TURNIPS	0.0
VEGETABLE JUICE	0.0
VEGETABLES (MIXED)	0.0
WATER CHESTNUTS	0.0
WHEAT FLOUR (ALL-PURPOSE, SIFTED	0.4
WHEAT FLOUR (ALL-PURPOSE, UNSIFTED)	0.3
WHOLE-WHEAT FLOUR	0.6
YOGURT (NONFAT MILK)	0.0

EAT FOODS FROM THIS TABLE AND FROM GREEN TABLE TWO FOR ONE WEEK THEN SWITCH TO 'YELLOW' TABLE ONE (DURING WEIGHT MAINTENANCE PHASE). ALSO CHOOSE ISOLATED ITEMS FROM THIS TABLE TO MAKE A BALANCED DIET WITH ANY ITEMS IN 'GREEN' TABLE TWO.

The Plateau-proof Diet '<u>Yellow</u>' Rotation Two Table (FP values)

APPLES (RAW, UNPEELED)	4.5
APPLESAUCE (CANNED,UNSWEETENED)	4.5
APRICOT (CANNED, HEAVY SYRUP)	2.5
APRICOT NECTAR	2.5
APRICOTS (CANNED, IN JUICE)	2.5
BAGELS (EGG)	3.8
BAGELS (PLAIN)	3.8
BAMBOO SHOOTS (CANNED)	2.3
BANANAS	4.5
BASS	2.7
BEER (LIGHT)	2.5
BEER (REGULAR)	2.5
BLACKBERRIES (RAW)	4.5
BLUE WHITING	2.9
BLUEBERRIES (RAW)	4.5
BOSTON BROWN BREAD	2.3
BOUILLON (DEHYDRATED)	4.5
BREADCRUMBS	4.3
BRILL	2.7
CANTALOUP	2.3
CARP	2.3
CATFISH	3.3
CATSUP	3.4
CELERY SEED	4.5
CHERRIES (RAW, SWEET)	4.5
CHESTNUTS (ROASTED)	2.7
CLAM CHOWDER (MANHATTAN, NO MILK)	2.3
CLUB SODA	4.5

COCKLE	3.4
COCOA POWDER (NONFAT DRY MILK)	4.0
COFFEE	4.5
COLA (DIET)	4.5
CORN (RAW, YELLOW)	2.3
CORNMEAL	2.0
CRACKED-WHEAT BREAD	2.3
CRANBERRY JUICE COCKTAL	4.5
CUCUMBER (WITH PEEL)	4.5
DANDELION GREENS	2.3
EGGS (HARD-BOILED)	3.9
EGGS (POACHED)	3.9
EGGS (SCRAMBLED)	4.7
EGGS (WHOLE, RAW)	3.9
ENGLISH MUFFINS (PLAIN)	3.4
FISH STICKS	2.3
FRENCH BREAD	4.6
FRUIT COCKTAIL (CANNED, JUICE)	2.5
GRAPE JUICE (CANNED)	2.5
GRAPEFRUIT JUICE (UNSWEETENED)	2.5
GRAPES (RAW)	4.5
GREY MULLET	4.2
HADDOCK (BREADED, FRIED)	2.6
ITALIAN BREAD	3.0
ITALIAN SALAD DRESSING (LOW CAL)	4.5
LEMON JUICE	4.5
LING	2.4
LIQUOR (GIN, RUM, VODKA, WHISKY, COGNAC...)	4.5
LOBSTER (BROWN MEAT)	2.5
MANGO (RAW)	4.5
MELBA TOAST	2.5
MINESTRONE SOUP	3.4
MISO	2.2
MIXED GRAIN BREAD	4.3
MUSSEL	2.1
MUSTARD (YELLOW)	4.5
NECTARINES	4.5
NORWAY POUT	2.8

OATMEAL (PLAIN)	2.3
OATMEAL BREAD	2.5
ORANGE & GRAPEFRUIT JUICE	2.5
ORANGE JUICE (CANNED, UNSWEETENED)	2.5
ORANGE JUICE (FRESH, UNSWEETENED)	2.5
OYSTER	2.3
PANCAKES (BUCKWHEAT)	4.5
PEACHES (CANNED, JUICE)	2.5
PEAR (CANNED, JUICE)	2.5
PEAR (FRESH)	4.5
PICKLES (CUCUMBER)	4.5
PICKLES (CUCUMBER, DILL)	4.5
PINEAPPLE (CANNED, JUICE)	2.5
PINEAPPLE (FRESH)	4.5
PINEAPPLE JUICE (UNSWEETENED)	2.5
PITA BREAD	3.3
PLUMS (CANNED, JUICE)	2.5
POLLACK	2.7
POPCORN (AIR-POPPED)	2.5
PRETZELS	4.8
PRUNE JUICE	2.5
PUMPERNICKEL BREAD	4.4
RADISHES	4.5
RAISIN BRAN CEREAL	4.0
RAISIN BREAD	4.8
RICE (WHITE)	2.5
ROLLS (HARD)	4.3
RYE BREAD (LIGHT)	2.2
RYE WAFERS (WHOLE-GRAIN)	4.5
SALMON (SMOKED)	4.5
SALTINES	4.5
SARDINES (CANNED, VEG OIL, ATLANTIC)	2.2
SCALLOPS (BREADED)	3.2
SEAWEED (KELP)	4.5
SELF-RISING FLOUR (UNSIFTED)	2.9
SHREDDED WHEAT CEREAL	4.0
SHRIMP (FRIED, NOT BREADED, NOT BATTERED)	3.0
SOYBEANS	2.4

SPECIAL K CEREAL (LOW-CARB)	2.5
SPRAT	2.0
SQUASH (SUMMER)	2.3
SQUASH (WINTER)	2.3
STRAWBERRIES (FRESH)	4.5
TANGERINE JUICE	2.5
TANGERINES (CANNED, LIGHT SYRUP)	2.5
TEA (BREWED, UNSWEETENED)	4.5
TOFU	2.5
TOMATO & VEGETABLE SOUP	4.5
TOMATO JUICE	2.5
TOMATO PUREE	2.5
TOMATO SOUP (WATER)	4.5
TOMATOES (CANNED)	2.3
TORTILLAS (CORN)	2.3
TROUT	4.6
VEGETARIAN SOUP	4.5
VIENNA BREAD	4.8
WATERMELON	3.0
WHEAT BREAD	2.2
WHEAT CRACKERS	4.5

AVOID THE FOODS IN THIS TABLE DURING THIS ROTATION

The Plateau-proof Diet '<u>Red</u>' Rotation Two Table (FP values)

ALMONDS (SLIVERED)	11.8
AMERICAN CHEESE	38.6
AMERICAN CHEESE SPREAD	34.2
ANGELFOOD CAKE	5.2
ANGLER	7.8
APPLE JUICE (CANNED)	7.0
APPLE PIE	30.9
APPLE PIE (FRIED)	41.7
APPLESAUCE (CANNED, SWEETENED)	9.5
AVOCADOS (CALIFORNIA)	33.9
AVOCADOS (FLORIDA)	24.5
BARBECUE SAUCE	7.0
BEAN WITH BACON SOUP	23.5
BEANS (CANNED, FRANKFURTER)	29.8
BEANS (PORK, SWEET SAUCE)	27.2
BEANS (PORK, TOMATO SAUCE)	24.5
BEEF (DRIED)	13.3
BEEF (LEAN & FAT CHUCK BLADE)	21.3
BEEF (LEAN & FAT, BOTTOM ROUND)	16.5
BEEF (LEAN, BOTTOM ROUND)	14.1
BEEF (LEAN, CHUCK BLADE)	16.9
BEEF AND VEGETABLE STEW	17.6
BEEF BROTH (BOULLION)	11.5
BEEF GRAVY	17.7
BEEF HEART (BRAISED)	11.0
BEEF LIVER (FRIED)	14.1
BEEF NOODLE SOUP	12.7
BEEF POTPIE	19.4
BEEF ROAST (LEAN, EYE O RND)	11.2
BEEF ROAST (LEAN & FAT, EYE O RND)	17.1
BEEF ROAST (LEAN & FAT, RIBS)	22.2
BEEF ROAST (LEAN, RIBS)	16.5

BEEF STEAK (LEAN, SIRLOIN, BROIL)	14.8
BISCUIT BAKING MIX	9.3
BLUE CHEESE	37.6
BLUE CHEESE SALAD DRESSING	56.1
BLUEBERRIES (FROZEN, SWEETENED)	5.0
BLUEBERRY MUFFINS	10.1
BLUEBERRY PIE	28.2
BOLOGNA	35.0
BRAN MUFFINS	6.1
BRAUNSCHWEIGER	34.2
BRAZIL NUTS	21.6
BREAD STUFFING (DRY MIX)	15.7
BROWN GRAVY (DRY MIX)	13.0
BROWNIES WITH NUTS	32.1
BUTTER	449.6
BUTTERMILK (DRIED)	29.7
BUTTERMILK (LIQUID)	21.5
CAKE & PASTRY FLOUR	5.6
CAMEMBERT CHEESE	36.5
CANDY (MILK CHOCOLATE, ALMONDS)	46.1
CANDY (MILK CHOCOLATE, PEANUTS)	41.5
CANDY (MILK CHOCOLATE, PLAIN)	54.9
CANDY (MILK CHOCOLATE, RICE CRISPIES)	50.2
CAP'N CRUNCH CEREAL	16.5
CARAMEL	20.2
CARROT CAKE (CREME CHESE FROSTING)	30.9
CASHEW NUTS (DRY ROASTD)	14.8
CASHEW NUTS (ROASTED, OIL)	13.7
CEREAL (100% NATURAL)	19.7
CHEDDAR CHEESE	38.3
CHEERIOS CEREAL	7.3
CHEESE CRACKERS (PEANUT SANDWICH)	31.5
CHEESE CRACKERS (PLAIN)	27.0
CHEESE SAUCE WITH MILK	34.3
CHEESEBURGER	34.2
CHEESECAKE	54.7
CHERRY PIE	27.7
CHERRY PIE (FRIED)	41.7

CHICKEN (CANNED)	21.8
CHICKEN (LIGHT & DARK, STEWED)	11.3
CHICKEN A LA KING	21.3
CHICKEN AND NOODLES	16.6
CHICKEN BREAST (FRIED, BATTERED)	17.6
CHICKEN BREAST (FRIED, FLOUR)	14.0
CHICKEN BREAST (ROASTED)	10.5
CHICKEN CHOW MEIN	10.0
CHICKEN DRUMSTICK (FRIED, BATTERED)	18.0
CHICKEN DRUMSTICK (ROASTED)	10.8
CHICKEN DRUMSTICK, (FRIED, FLOUR)	15.1
CHICKEN FRANKFURTER	27.0
CHICKEN GRAVY (CANNED)	22.8
CHICKEN GRAVY (DRY MIX)	13.0
CHICKEN LIVER	10.9
CHICKEN NOODLE SOUP	12.3
CHICKEN POTPIE	23.1
CHICKEN RICE SOUP	12.3
CHICKEN ROLL	14.3
CHILI	8.1
CHOCOLATE (SWEET, DARK)	79.6
CHOCOLATE (FOR BAKING, BITTER)	33.9
CHOCOLATE CHIP COOKIES	28.0
CHOCOLATE MILK (LOWFAT 1%)	26.9
CHOCOLATE MILK (LOWFAT 2%)	35.0
CHOCOLATE MILK (REGULAR)	40.7
CHOCOLATE PUDDING	34.3
CHOCOLATE SHAKE	38.5
CHOP SUEY (BEEF & PORK)	15.5
CHOW MEIN NOODLES	8.4
CLAM CHOWDER (NEW ENGLAND, MILK)	27.5
COCOA POWDER (REGULAR)	34.1
COCONUT (RAW)	115.2
COCONUT (SHREDDED, DRIED, SWEETENED)	114.7
COFFEE CREAM (LIGHT)	69.8
COFFEECAKE (CRUMB)	15.4
COLA (REGULAR)	9.5
CONDENSED MILK (SWEETENED)	44.2

CONGER	6.5
CORN CHIPS	20.3
CORN FLAKES	5.0
CORN MUFFINS	7.6
CORN OIL	981000.1
CORNED BEEF (CANNED)	26.7
COTTAGE CHEESE (FRUIT)	31.2
COTTAGE CHEESE (LARGE CURDS, CREAMED)	33.3
COTTAGE CHEESE (LOWFAT 2%)	28.8
COTTAGE CHEESE (UNCREAMED)	20.2
CRAB (BROWN MEAT)	7.2
CRAB (WHITE MEAT)	9.0
CRACKERS (SNACK)	4502.5
CRANBERRY SAUCE (SWEATENED, CANNED)	5.0
CREAM CHEESE	53.3
CREAM OF CHICKEN SOUP (MILK)	32.0
CREAM OF CHICKEN SOUP (WATER)	20.7
CREAM OF MUSHROM SOUP (MILK)	34.6
CREAM OF MUSHROOM SOUP (WATER)	20.4
CREAM OF WHEAT	5.0
CREME PIE	54.2
CROISSANTS	15.9
CUSTARD (BAKED)	14.0
CUSTARD PIE	16.0
DANISH PASTRY (FRUIT)	22.5
DANISH PASTRY (PLAIN)	24.3
DEVIL'S FOOD CAKE (CHOCOLATE FROSTING)	25.3
DOGFISH	5.2
DOUGHNUTS (CAKE TYPE, PLAIN)	23.2
DOUGHNUTS (YEAST-LEAVENED, GLAZED)	29.3
DUCK (ROASTED)	17.2
EEL	22.7
EGG NOG	21.3
EGGS (FRIED)	5.4
EGGS (YOLK, RAW)	7.6
ENCHILADA	10.8
ENG MUFFIN (BACON, EGG, CHEESE)	33.4
EVAPORATED MILK (WHOLE)	37.6

FETA CHEESE	38.2
FIG BARS	11.5
FILBERTS (HAZELNUTS)	21.7
FISH SANDWICH (CHEESE)	32.0
FISH SANDWICH (NO CHEESE)	11.7
FLOUNDER (BAKED IN BUTTER)	27.5
FRANKFURTER	35.8
FRENCH SALAD DRESSING (LOW CAL)	9005.0
FRENCH SALAD DRESSING (REGULAR)	40505.0
FRENCH TOAST	7.8
FROOT LOOPS CEREAL	7.3
FROSTED FLAKES CEREAL	5.0
FRUIT COCKTAIL (CANNED, HEAVY SYRUP)	5.0
FRUIT JELLIES	9.5
FRUIT PUNCH DRINK (CANNED)	9.5
FRUITCAKE	21.5
FUDGE, CHOCOLATE, PLAIN	25.5
GELATIN DESSERT	5.0
GINGER ALE	9.5
GINGERBREAD CAKE	15.1
GOLDEN GRAHAMS CEREAL	7.3
GRAHAM CRACKER (PLAIN)	7.0
GRAPE DRINK (CANNED)	9.5
GRAPE SODA	9.5
GRAPEFRUIT (CANNED, SYRUP)	5.0
GRAPEFRUIT JUICE (SWEETENED)	5.0
GRAPE-NUTS CEREAL	5.0
GROUND BEEF (BROILED, LEAN & FAT)	19.0
GROUND BEEF (BROILED, LEAN)	18.2
GUM DROPS	9.5
HALF AND HALF (CREAM)	51.9
HALIBUT	5.5
HALIBUT (BROILED, BUTTER & LEMON JUICE)	7.6
HAMBURGER	21.1
HARD CANDY	9.5
HERRING	12.4
HERRING (PICKLED)	6.8
HOLLANDAISE (WATER)	49.3

HONEY	5.0
HONEY NUT CHEERIOS CEREAL	6.5
ICE CREAM (VANLLA,11% FAT)	54.3
ICE CREAM (VANLLA,16% FAT)	67.0
ICE MILK (VANILLA, 3%)	33.9
ICE MILK (VANILLA, 4% FAT)	45.0
IMITATION CREAMER (POWDERED)	4520.0
IMITATION SOUR DRESSING	76.2
IMITATION WHIPPED TOPING	3620.0
ITALIAN SALAD DRESSING (REGULAR)	40500.0
JAMS AND FRUIT PRESERVES	7.0
JELLY BEANS	9.5
JOHN DORY	14.6
LAMB (LEG, LEAN & FAT, ROASTED)	18.2
LAMB (LEG, LEAN, ROASTED)	14.4
LAMB CHOPS (ARM, LEAN & FAT, BRAISED)	19.9
LAMB CHOPS (ARM, LEAN, BRAISED)	15.7
LAMB CHOPS (LOIN, LEAN & FAT, BROIL)	19.8
LAMB CHOPS (LOIN, LEAN, BROIL)	15.0
LAMB RIB (LEAN & FAT, ROASTED)	23.9
LAMB RIB (LEAN, ROASTED)	16.7
LARD	922526.3
LEMON MERINGUE PIE	16.6
LEMONADE	9.5
LEMON-LIME SODA	9.5
LOBSTER (WHITE MEAT)	16.8
LUCKY CHARMS CEREAL	6.5
MACADAMIA NUTS (OIL ROASTED)	46.5
MACARONI AND CHEESE	32.5
MALTED MILK (CHOCOLATE)	39.5
MALTED MILK (REGULAR)	39.1
MALT-O-MEAL	25.0
MARGARINE (REGULAR, HARD)	49500.1
MARGARINE (IMITATION 40% FAT)	396.2
MARGARINE (REGULAR, HARD, 80% FAT)	409.7
MARGARINE (REGULR, SOFT)	49500.1
MARGARINE (REGULR, SOFT, 80% FAT)	823.7
MARGARINE (SPREAD, HARD, 60% FAT)	313.3

MARGARINE (SPREAD, SOFT, 60% FAT)	623.6
MARSHMALLOWS	5.0
MAYONNAISE (IMITATION)	13520.0
MAYONNAISE (REGULAR)	49520.1
MAYONNAISE SALAD DRESSING	22520.0
MEGRIM	13.5
MILK (1% LOW FAT)	24.4
MILK (2% LOW FAT)	28.6
MILK (WHOLE)	35.0
MIXED NUTS (DRY ROASTED, NO HONEY)	16.9
MIXED NUTS (OIL ROASTED, NO HONEY)	14.5
MOLASSES	9.5
MOZZARELLA CHEESE (WHOLE MILK)	32.7
MOZZARELLA CHESE (NONFAT MILK)	10.0
MUENSTER CHEESE	35.4
MUSHROOM GRAVY	19.0
NATURE VALLEY GRANOLA CEREAL	21.0
OATMEAL & RAISIN COOKIES	20.2
OCEAN PERCH (FRIED, BREADED)	5.8
OLIVE OIL	972000.2
OLIVES (BLACK)	9000.0
OLIVES (GREEN)	9000.0
ONION RINGS	25.2
ORANGE SODA	9.5
OYSTERS (FRIED, BREADED)	7.1
PANCAKES (PLAIN)	7.0
PARMESAN CHEESE	38.4
PARMESAN CHEESE	33.3
PEACH PIE	26.9
PEACHES (CANNED, HEAVY SYRUP)	5.0
PEANUT BUTTER	7.3
PEANUT BUTTER COOKIE	23.5
PEANUT OIL	972000.2
PEANUTS (OIL-ROASTED)	7.9
PEAR (CANNED, HEAVY SYRUP)	5.0
PECAN PIE	27.7
PECANS (HALVES)	41.1
PERCH	5.3

PICKLES (CUCUMBER, SWEET)	9.5
PIE CRUST	26.4
PILCHARD (S. AFRICAN)	10.9
PINE NUTS	38.4
PINEAPPLE (CANNED, HEAVY SYRUP)	5.0
PINEAPPLE-GRAPEFRUIT JUICE DRINK	9.5
PISTACHIO NUTS	10.6
PIZZA (CHEESE)	30.7
PLAICE	9.5
PLUMS (CANNED, HEAVY SYRUP)	5.0
POPCORN (SYRUP)	7.3
POPCORN (VEGETABLE OIL)	16.0
POPSICLE	9.5
PORK (CURED, BACON)	20.2
PORK (CURED, CANADIAN BACON)	11.7
PORK (CURED, HAM, LEAN & FAT)	17.8
PORK (CURED, HAM, LEAN)	11.1
PORK (LINK)	16.1
PORK (LUNCHEON MEAT, CANNED)	25.4
PORK (LUNCHEON MEAT, HAM, LEAN & FAT)	12.9
PORK (LUNCHEON MEAT, HAM, LEAN)	11.2
PORK (ROASTED HAM, LEAN)	14.5
PORK CHOP LOIN (BROILED, LEAN & FAT)	18.3
PORK CHOP LOIN (BROILED, LEAN)	14.1
PORK CHOP LOIN (FRIED, LEAN & FAT)	20.6
PORK CHOP LOIN (FRIED, LEAN)	16.1
PORK FRESH (ROASTED HAM, LEAN & FAT)	18.4
PORK RIBS (ROASTED, LEAN & FAT)	18.8
PORK RIBS (ROASTED, LEAN)	15.5
PORK SHOULDER (BRAISED, LEAN & FAT)	18.9
PORK SHOULDER (BRAISED, LEAN)	14.5
POTATO CHIPS	31.6
POTATO SALAD (MAYONNAISE)	33.6
POTATOES (AU GRATIN)	40.3
POTATOES (FRENCH FRIES, BAKED)	12.8
POTATOES (FRENCH FRIES, FRIED)	18.2
POTATOES (HASHED BROWN)	21.2
POTATOES (MASHED)	24.2

POTATOES (SCALLOPED)	39.9
POUND CAKE	33.2
PRODUCT 19 CEREAL	5.0
PROVOLONE CHEESE	34.1
PUMPKIN AND SQUASH KERNELS	8.5
PUMPKIN PIE	23.8
QUICHE LORRAINE	47.7
RASPBERRIES (SWEETENED)	5.0
RED MULLET	6.2
RELISH (SWEET)	9.5
RHUBARB (SWEETENED)	5.0
RICE KRISPIES CEREAL	5.0
RICE PUDDING	34.3
RICOTTA CHEESE (NONFAT MILK)	17.2
RICOTTA CHEESE (WHOLE MILK)	40.5
ROAST BEEF SANDWICH	17.6
ROLLS (FOR FRANKFURTER & HAMBURGER)	5.5
ROLLS (DINNER)	11.5
ROLLS (FOR HOAGIE OR SUBMARINE)	5.9
ROOT BEER	9.5
SAFFLOWER OIL	981000.1
SAITHE	5.5
SALAMI (DRY)	28.8
SALAMI (NOT DRY)	31.1
SALMON (PACIFIC)	74.2
SAND EEL	7.2
SANDWICH SPREAD (BEEF & PORK)	23.5
SAUSAGE (BROWN AND SERVE)	31.4
SEA BREAM	7.5
SEMI SWEET CHOCOLATE	77.8
SESAME SEEDS	9.0
SHEETCAKE (NO FROSTING)	23.3
SHEETCAKE (WHITE FROSTING)	29.5
SHERBET	47.0
SHORTBREAD COOKIE	199.5
SNACK CAKES (DEVIL'S FOOD & CRÈME)	25.1
SNACK CAKES (SPONGE & CRÈME)	31.0
SOLE (BAKED IN BUTTER)	27.5

SOUR CREAM	66.2
SOYBEAN OIL (HYDROGENATED)	981000.2
SOYBEAN-COTTONSEED OIL (HYDROGENATED)	981000.2
SPAGHETTI (MEATBALLS, TOMATO SAUCE)	13.9
SPAGHETTI (TOMATO SAUCE, CHEESE)	21.5
SPINACH SOUFFLE	32.5
STEAK (BROILED, SIRLOIN)	18.5
STRAWBERRIES (FROZEN, SWEETENED)	9.5
SUGAR (BROWN)	9.5
SUGAR (WHITE)	9.5
SUGAR COOKIE	32.1
SUGAR SMACKS CEREAL	7.3
SUNFLOWER OIL	981000.1
SUNFLOWER SEEDS	10.5
SUPER SUGAR CRISP CEREAL	5.0
SWEET POTATOE PIE	13505.2
SWISS CHEESE	34.5
SWISS CHEESE	34.5
SYRUP (LIGHT, CHOCOLATE FLAVORED)	5.0
SYRUP (CORN, MAPLE)	9.5
SYRUP (THICK, CHOCOLATE FLAVORED)	23.5
TACO	9.4
TAHINI	12.0
TAPIOCA PUDDING	64.2
TARTAR SAUCE	36000.0
THOUSAND ISLAND DRESSING	27000.0
TOASTER PASTRIES	18.6
TOMATO SOUP (MILK)	29.1
TOTAL CEREAL	6.5
TRIX CEREAL	5.0
TROUT (BROILED, BUTTER)	27.2
TUNA	9.8
TUNA SALAD	22.7
TURBOT	14.4
TURKEY (LIGHT & DARK, ROASTED)	11.0
TURKEY (ROASTED)	10.5
TURKEY AND GRAVY	12.6
TURKEY HAM (CURED)	11.2

TURKEY LOAF	10.5
TURKEY PATTIES (BATTERED, FRIED)	18.0
TUSK	6.5
VANILLA PUDDING	104.2
VANILLA SHAKE	37.8
VANILLA WAFERS	20.9
VEAL CUTLET (BROILED, ROASTED, BRAISED)	17.1
VEAL RIB (BROILED, ROASTED, BRAISED)	18.3
VEGETABLE & BEEF SOUP	11.5
VIENNA SAUSAGE	29.1
VINEGAR AND OIL SALAD DRESSING	36000.1
WAFFLES	10.3
WALNUTS (BLACK)	10.3
WALNUTS (ENGLISH)	19.7
WHEATIES CEREAL	5.0
WHIPPED TOPPING	67.1
WHIPPING CREAM (HEAVY)	119.9
WHIPPING CREAM (LIGHT)	107.3
WHITE BREAD	10.6
WHITE BREAD CRUMBS	7.3
WHITE BREAD CUBES	7.3
WHITE CAKE (WHITE FROSTING)	23.3
WHITE SAUCE (MILK)	33.0
WHOLE-WHEAT BREAD	5.3
WHOLE-WHEAT WAFERS	9.0
YELLOW CAKE (CHOCOLATE FROSTING)	43.8
YOGURT (FRUIT, LOW FAT MILK)	25.2
YOGURT (PLAIN, LOW FAT MILK)	26.3
YOGURT (WHOLE MILK)	35.8

The Plateau-proof Diet <u>Turbo</u> for Hypertension – The weight loss solution for stubborn obesity

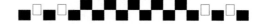

It is more difficult for people with hypertension and associated conditions such as type II diabetes to lose weight, compared to normotensive (non-hypertensive) obese individuals. The plateau-proof diet for hypertension is designed to effectively affect weight loss in overweight and obese individuals with hypertension. Most patients with hypertension will find the plateau-proof diet for hypertension adequate for an efficient and sustainable weight loss. The most stubborn weight gain cases; however, cannot be ignored. Typically these cases are unresponsive to dietary weight loss therapy and to exercise. For these cases, the plateau-proof diet for hypertension has been modified to the plateau-proof diet turbo for hypertension.

The plateau-proof diet turbo for hypertension is designed to affect weight loss in the most stubborn cases of obesity. The diet is the same as the plateau-proof diet for hypertension, except that the perfect cardio index (PCi) is doubled in the turbo diet. <u>The effect of doubling the PCi is the exclusion of meats and many animal products from the diet. The exclusion of meats lowers saturated fats and iron, both of which have been implicated in the etiology of hypertension and the commonly associated type II diabetes.</u> The exclusion of animal products lowers saturated fats. The rationale is to return hypertensive individuals to metabolic stability as fast as possible, facilitating later weight loss. It has been shown that decreasing the amount of iron in the blood improves the symptoms of hypertension and type II diabetes. It has also been shown that decreasing the amount of saturated fats in the diet improves blood lipid profiles and improves the symptoms of hypertension and type II diabetes. Improving the symptoms of hypertension and type II diabetes from metabolic control and weight loss should facilitate further weight loss in the stubborn cases of obesity. Further weight loss should lead to increased metabolic stability, which in turn should facilitate weight loss.

The plateau-proof diet turbo for hypertension has the same CP and FP formulas as the plateau-proof diet for hypertension, except that the PCi is doubled in the CP and FP formulas in the turbo diet. The instructions for using the plateau-proof diet turbo are the same as the instructions for the plateau-proof diet for hypertension in the previous chapter.

EAT FOODS FROM THIS TABLE FOR 4 WEEKS THEN SWITCH TO 'GREEN' TABLE TWO (DURING WEIGHT LOSS PHASE)

The Plateau-proof Turbo '<u>Green</u>' Rotation One Table (CP values)

ALFALFA SEEDS (SPROUTED, RAW)	1.5
ALMONDS (SLIVERED)	1.6
ANGLER	0.0
ASPARAGUS (CANNED)	3.0
ASPARAGUS (FROZEN)	1.5
BAMBOO SHOOTS (CANNED)	3.0
BASS	0.0
BEAN SPROUTS	2.5
BEET GREENS	3.0
BLACK BEANS (COOKED, DRAINED)	1.4
BLACK-EYED PEAS, DRY, COOKED	1.5
BLUE WHITING	0.0
BOUILLON (DEHYDRATED)	2.0
BRAZIL NUTS	1.5
BRILL	0.0
BROCCOLI (FROZEN, COOKED, DRAINED)	1.7
BROCCOLI (RAW, COOKED, DRAINED)	2.3
BRUSSELS SPROUTS	3.3
CABBAGE (CHINESE)	1.5
CARP	0.0
CASHEW NUTS (DRY ROASTD)	4.5
CASHEW NUTS (ROASTED, VEG OIL)	3.5
CATFISH	0.0
CAULIFLOWER	4.5
CELERY (PASCAL, RAW)	2.0
CHICKPEAS	3.2
CHILI	2.4
CLAM CHOWDER (NEW ENGLAND, NONFAT MILK)	3.8
CLAMS	0.4
CLUB SODA	2.0
COCKLE	0.0

COD	0.0
COFFEE	2.0
COLA (DIET)	2.0
COLLARDS	3.8
CONGER	0.0
CORN OIL	2.0
CRAB (BROWN MEAT)	0.0
CRAB (WHITE MEAT)	0.0
CRABMEAT	0.1
CUSTARD (BAKED)	4.5
DAB	0.0
DOGFISH	0.0
EEL	0.0
ENCHILADA (Vegetable or seafood)	2.4
ENDIVE	4.0
EVAPORATED MILK (NONFAT)	3.1
FILBERTS (HAZELNUTS)	2.4
FISH SANDWICH (NO CHEESE)	4.6
FISH STICKS	1.3
FLOUNDER	0.0
FLOUNDER (BAKED WITH VEG OIL)	0.0
FLOUNDER (BAKED, NO FAT)	0.0
GREAT NORTHERN BEANS (DRY, DRAINED)	2.9
GREEN PEAS (SOUP)	4.5
GREY MULLET	0.0
GURNARD	0.0
HADDOCK	0.0
HADDOCK (BREADED, FRIED)	0.8
HAKE	0.0
HAKE (S. AFRICAN)	0.0
HALIBUT	0.0
HALIBUT (BROILED, LEMON JUICE)	0.0
HERRING	0.0
HERRING (PICKLED)	0.0
JOHN DORY	0.0
KALE	3.5
KING CRAB (WHITE MEAT)	0.0
LEMON SOLE	0.0

LENTILS	1.2
LETTUCE (BUTTER-HEAD)	4.0
LETTUCE (CRISP-HEAD)	4.4
LETTUCE (LOOSE LEAF)	4.0
LIMA BEANS	3.1
LING	0.0
LIQUOR (GIN, RUM, VODKA, WHISKY, COGNAC...)	2.0
LOBSTER (BROWN MEAT)	0.0
LOBSTER (WHITE MEAT)	0.0
MACADAMIA NUTS (VEG OIL-ROASTED)	3.4
MACKEREL	0.0
MEGRIM	0.0
MILK (NONFAT)	2.7
MISO	4.6
MIXED NUTS (DRY ROASTED, NO HONEY)	2.6
MIXED NUTS (VEG OIL-ROASTED, NO HONEY)	1.8
MUSSEL	0.0
MUSTARD (YELLOW)	2.0
MUSTARD GREENS	2.0
NONFAT DRY MILK	3.0
NORWAY LOBSTER (WHITE MEAT)	0.0
NORWAY POUT	0.0
OCEAN PERCH (FRIED IN VEG OIL, BREADED)	0.9
OKRA	4.5
OLIVE OIL	2.0
OLIVES (BLACK)	2.0
OLIVES (GREEN)	2.0
ONIONS (RAW, SPRING)	4.0
OYSTER	0.0
OYSTERS (FRIED, BREADED)	2.0
OYSTERS (RAW)	0.8
PEA BEANS (DRY)	4.0
PEANUT BUTTER	1.2
PEANUT OIL	2.0
PEANUTS (VEG OIL-ROASTED)	1.3
PEAS (FRESH, GREEN)	4.3
PEAS (POD)	3.3
PECANS (HALVES)	5.0

PERCH	0.0
PILCHARD	0.0
PILCHARD (S. AFRICAN)	0.0
PINE NUTS	5.0
PINTO BEANS	4.9
PISTACHIO NUTS	1.8
PLAICE	0.0
POLLACK	0.0
PRAWN	0.0
PUMPKIN AND SQUASH KERNELS	1.4
RED KIDNEY BEANS	2.8
RED MULLET	0.0
REDFISH	0.0
REFRIED BEANS	4.3
RICOTTA CHEESE (NONFAT MILK)	0.9
SAFFLOWER OIL	2.0
SAITHE	0.0
SALMON	0.0
SALMON (CANNED)	0.0
SALMON (PACIFIC)	0.0
SALMON (RED, BAKED)	0.0
SALMON (SMOKED)	0.0
SAND EEL	0.0
SARDINES (CANNED, VEG OIL, ATLANTIC)	0.0
SCALLOP	0.0
SCALLOPS (BREADED)	1.3
SEA BREAM	0.0
SEAWEED (SPIRULINA)	0.9
SESAME SEEDS	1.0
SHRIMP	0.0
SHRIMP	0.1
SHRIMP (FRIED VEG OIL, NOT BREADED / BATTERED)	1.4
SKATE RAY	0.0
SNAP BEAN (GREEN)	4.5
SNAP BEAN (YELLOW)	4.5
SOLE	0.0
SOLE (BAKED, NO FAT)	0.0
SOY SAUCE	2.0

SOYBEAN OIL	2.0
SOYBEAN-COTTONSEED OIL	2.0
SOYBEANS	1.5
SPAGHETTI (MEATBALLS, TOMATO SAUCE)	4.8
SPINACH (CANNED)	1.8
SPINACH (FRESH)	1.5
SPINACH (FROZEN)	2.5
SPRAT	0.0
SQUID	0.0
SUNFLOWER OIL	2.0
SUNFLOWER SEEDS	1.7
TACO	3.3
TAHINI	2.0
TEA (BREWED, UNSWEETENED)	2.0
TOFU	0.7
TROUT	0.0
TROUT (BROILED)	0.0
TUNA	0.0
TUNA (CANNED, LIGHT, VEG OIL, DRAINNED)	0.0
TUNA (CANNED, LIGHT, WATER)	0.0
TURBOT	0.0
TURNIP GREENS (FROZEN)	3.2
TUSK	0.0
VINEGAR AND OIL SALAD DRESSING	2.0
WALNUTS (BLACK)	0.6
WALNUTS (ENGLISH)	1.9
WHITE SAUCE (NONFAT MILK)	4.2
YOGURT (NONFAT MILK)	2.8

EAT FOODS FROM THIS TABLE AND FROM 'GREEN' TABLE ONE FOR 4 WEEKS THEN SWITCH TO 'YELLOW' TABLE TWO (DURING WEIGHT MAINTENANCE PHASE). ALSO CHOOSE ISOLATED ITEMS FROM THIS TABLE TO MAKE A BALANCED DIET WITH ANY ITEMS IN 'GREEN' TABLE ONE.

The Plateau-proof Turbo 'Yellow' Rotation One Table (CP values)

ALL-BRAN CEREAL	5.3
ARTICHOKES (GLOBE, COOKED)	6.0
AVOCADOS (CALIFORNIA)	6.0
BEER (LIGHT)	10.0
CABBAGE (RED)	6.0
CABBAGE (SAVOY)	6.0
CARROTS (FROZEN, COOKED)	9.0
CELERY SEED	10.0
CEREAL (100% NATURAL)	6.0
CHEERIOS CEREAL	10.0
CHOW MEIN NOODLES	8.7
CLAM CHOWDER (MANHATTAN)	6.0
CORN (RAW, WHITE)	9.5
CREAM OF MUSHROOM SOUP (WATER)	9.0
CUSTARD PIE	8.2
DANDELION GREENS	5.3
KOHLRABI	7.3
LEMONS (RAW)	10.0
MELBA TOAST	8.0
MINESTRONE SOUP	5.5
MIXED GRAIN BREAD	9.4
MUSHROOMS (CANNED)	5.3
MUSHROOMS (RAW)	6.0
OATMEAL (PLAIN)	9.0
ONION SOUP	8.0
PEAS (CANNED, GREEN)	5.3
PEPPERS (HOT GREEN CHILI)	8.0
PEPPERS (HOT RED CHILI)	8.0

PEPPERS (SWEET GREEN)	8.0
PEPPERS (SWEET RED)	8.0
POPCORN (AIR-POPPED)	9.0
POPCORN (VEGETABLE OIL)	9.0
RYE BREAD (LIGHT)	8.6
SAUERKRAUT	7.5
SPAGHETTI (FIRM)	8.4
SPECIAL K CEREAL (LOW-CARB)	7.0
SQUASH (SUMMER)	8.0
TOMATO JUICE	10.0
TOMATO SOUP (NONFAT MILK)	7.3
TOMATOES (CANNED)	10.0
TOMATOES (FRESH)	7.5
TORTILLAS (CORN)	9.8
TURNIP GREENS (FRESH)	6.0
VEGETABLE JUICE	8.3
VEGETABLES (MIXED)	5.6
VEGETARIAN SOUP	9.0
WAFFLES	7.7
WHEAT CRACKERS	10.0
WHIPPED TOPPING	7.0
WHOLE-WHEAT BREAD	7.2
WHOLE-WHEAT FLOUR	8.0
WHOLE-WHEAT WAFERS	7.5

AVOID THE FOODS IN THIS TABLE DURING THIS ROTATION

The Plateau-proof Turbo '<u>Red</u>' Rotation One Table (CP values)

AMERICAN CHEESE	40.0
AMERICAN CHEESE SPREAD	40.8
ANGELFOOD CAKE	18.0
APPLE JUICE (CANNED)	58000.0
APPLE PIE	34.3
APPLE PIE (FRIED)	31.0
APPLES (RAW, UNPEELED)	480.0
APPLES (DRIED, SULFURED)	630.0
APPLESAUCE (CANNED, SWEETENED)	1020.0
APPLESAUCE (CANNED,UNSWEETENED)	560.0
APRICOT (CANNED, HEAVY SYRUP)	110.0
APRICOT NECTAR	72.0
APRICOTS (CANNED, IN JUICE)	31.0
APRICOTS (DRIED)	27.5
APRICOTS (RAW)	18.0
AVOCADOS (FLORIDA)	10.8
BAGELS (EGG)	10.9
BAGELS (PLAIN)	10.9
BANANAS	54.0
BARBECUE SAUCE	4000.0
BARLEY (PEARLED, LIGHT)	14.8
BEAN WITH BACON SOUP	22.9
BEANS (CANNED, FRANKFURTER)	21.7
BEANS (PORK, SWEET SAUCE)	23.4
BEANS (PORK, TOMATO SAUCE)	23.0
BEEF (DRIED)	20.0
BEEF (LEAN & FAT CHUCK BLADE)	20.0
BEEF (LEAN & FAT, BOTTOM ROUND)	20.0
BEEF (LEAN, BOTTOM ROUND)	20.0
BEEF (LEAN, CHUCK BLADE)	20.0
BEEF AND VEGETABLE STEW	21.4
BEEF BROTH (BOULLION)	20.0

BEEF GRAVY	22.4
BEEF HEART (BRAISED)	20.0
BEEF LIVER (FRIED)	20.6
BEEF NOODLE SOUP	23.6
BEEF POTPIE	23.7
BEEF ROAST (LEAN, EYE O RND)	20.0
BEEF ROAST (LEAN & FAT, EYE O RND)	20.0
BEEF ROAST (LEAN & FAT, RIBS)	20.0
BEEF ROAST (LEAN, RIBS)	20.0
BEEF STEAK (LEAN, SIRLOIN, BROIL)	20.0
BEER (REGULAR)	26.0
BEETS (CANNED)	12.0
BEETS (COOKED, DRAINED)	14.0
BISCUIT BAKING MIX	14.0
BLACKBERRIES (RAW)	27.0
BLUE CHEESE	40.3
BLUE CHEESE SALAD DRESSING	42.0
BLUEBERRIES (FROZEN, SWEETENED)	100.0
BLUEBERRIES (RAW)	40.0
BLUEBERRY MUFFINS	13.3
BLUEBERRY PIE	28.7
BOLOGNA	40.6
BOSTON BROWN BREAD	21.0
BRAN FLAKES (40%)	11.0
BRAN MUFFINS	12.0
BRAUNSCHWEIGER	40.5
BREAD STUFFING (DRY MIX)	11.1
BREADCRUMBS	11.2
BROWN GRAVY (DRY MIX)	29.3
BROWNIES WITH NUTS	22.0
BUCKWHEAT FLOUR (LIGHT, SIFTED)	19.5
BULGUR	13.6
BUTTER	40.0
BUTTERMILK (DRIED)	42.9
BUTTERMILK (LIQUID)	43.4
CABBAGE (COMMON)	10.5
CAKE & PASTRY FLOUR	21.7
CAMEMBERT CHEESE	40.0

CANDY (MILK CHOCOLATE, ALMONDS)	50.0
CANDY (MILK CHOCOLATE, PEANUTS)	46.5
CANDY (MILK CHOCOLATE, PLAIN)	56.0
CANDY (MILK CHOCOLATE, RICE CRISPIES)	58.0
CANTALOUP	22.0
CAP'N CRUNCH CEREAL	46.0
CARAMEL	44.0
CAROB FLOUR	42.0
CARROT CAKE (CREME CHESE FROSTING)	44.6
CARROTS (RAW)	12.0
CATSUP	27.6
CHEDDAR CHEESE	40.0
CHEESE CRACKERS (PEANUT SANDWICH)	30.0
CHEESE CRACKERS (PLAIN)	32.0
CHEESE SAUCE WITH MILK	42.9
CHEESEBURGER	43.7
CHEESECAKE	51.3
CHERRIES (RAW, SWEET)	22.0
CHERRIES (SOUR, CANNED, WATER)	44.0
CHERRY PIE	29.0
CHERRY PIE (FRIED)	32.0
CHESTNUTS (ROASTED)	30.4
CHICKEN (CANNED)	20.0
CHICKEN (LIGHT & DARK, STEWED)	20.0
CHICKEN A LA KING	20.9
CHICKEN AND NOODLES	22.4
CHICKEN BREAST (FRIED, BATTERED)	20.7
CHICKEN BREAST (FRIED, FLOUR)	20.1
CHICKEN BREAST (ROASTED)	20.0
CHICKEN CHOW MEIN	25.1
CHICKEN DRUMSTICK (FRIED, BATTERED)	20.8
CHICKEN DRUMSTICK (ROASTED)	20.0
CHICKEN DRUMSTICK, (FRIED, FLOUR)	20.2
CHICKEN FRANKFURTER	41.0
CHICKEN GRAVY (CANNED)	25.2
CHICKEN GRAVY (DRY MIX)	29.3
CHICKEN LIVER	20.0
CHICKEN NOODLE SOUP	24.5

CHICKEN POTPIE	23.8
CHICKEN RICE SOUP	23.5
CHICKEN ROLL	20.2
CHOCOLATE (SWEET, DARK)	72.0
CHOCOLATE (FOR BAKING, BITTER)	45.3
CHOCOLATE CHIP COOKIES	28.0
CHOCOLATE MILK (LOWFAT 1%)	46.5
CHOCOLATE MILK (LOWFAT 2%)	46.5
CHOCOLATE MILK (REGULAR)	46.5
CHOCOLATE PUDDING (nonfat milk)	13.5
CHOCOLATE SHAKE	55.0
CHOP SUEY (BEEF & PORK)	41.0
COCOA POWDER (NO FAT DRY MILK)	14.7
COCOA POWDER (REGULAR)	46.7
COCONUT (RAW)	10.5
COCONUT (SHREDDED, DRIED, SWEETENED)	22.0
COFFEE CREAM (LIGHT)	23.0
COFFEECAKE (CRUMB)	16.7
COLA (REGULAR)	82000.0
CONDENSED MILK (SWEETENED)	53.8
CORN (CREAM, CANNED)	23.0
CORN (RAW, YELLOW)	14.3
CORN CHIPS	16.0
CORN FLAKES	24.0
CORN GRITS (WHITE)	20.7
CORN GRITS (YELLOW)	20.7
CORN MUFFINS	14.0
CORNED BEEF (CANNED)	20.0
CORNMEAL	16.4
COTTAGE CHEESE (FRUIT)	42.9
COTTAGE CHEESE (LARGE CURDS, CREAMED)	40.4
COTTAGE CHEESE (LOWFAT 2%)	20.5
COTTAGE CHEESE (UNCREAMED)	40.2
CRACKED-WHEAT BREAD	12.0
CRACKED-WHEAT BREAD	10.8
CRACKERS (SNACK)	40.0
CRANBERRY JUICE COCKTAL	76000.0
CRANBERRY SAUCE (SWEATENED, CANNED)	216.0

CREAM CHEESE	41.0
CREAM OF CHICKEN SOUP (MILK)	44.3
CREAM OF CHICKEN SOUP (WATER)	26.0
CREAM OF MUSHROM SOUP (MILK)	45.0
CREAM OF WHEAT	14.0
CREME PIE	35.1
CROISSANTS	10.8
CUCUMBER (WITH PEEL)	200.0
DANISH PASTRY (FRUIT)	14.0
DANISH PASTRY (PLAIN)	14.5
DATES	32.8
DEVIL'S FOOD CAKE (CHOCOLATE FROSTING)	28.7
DOUGHNUTS (CAKE TYPE, PLAIN)	16.0
DOUGHNUTS (YEAST-LEAVENED, GLAZED)	17.3
DUCK (ROASTED)	20.0
EGG NOG	27.6
EGG NOODLES	10.6
EGGPLANT	12.0
EGGS (FRIED)	20.3
EGGS (HARD-BOILED)	20.3
EGGS (POACHED)	20.3
EGGS (SCRAMBLED)	20.3
EGGS (WHITE, RAW)	20.0
EGGS (WHOLE, RAW)	20.3
EGGS (YOLK, RAW)	20.0
ENG MUFFIN (BACON, EGG, CHEESE)	43.4
ENGLISH MUFFINS (PLAIN)	10.8
EVAPORATED MILK (WHOLE)	42.9
FETA CHEESE	40.5
FIG BARS	31.5
FIGS (DRIED)	20.3
FISH SANDWICH (CHEESE)	44.9
FLOUNDER (BAKED IN BUTTER)	40.0
FRANKFURTER	40.4
FRENCH BREAD	10.7
FRENCH SALAD DRESSING (LOW CAL)	4000.0
FRENCH SALAD DRESSING (REGULAR)	2000.0
FRENCH TOAST	25.7

FROOT LOOPS CEREAL	25.0
FROSTED FLAKES CEREAL	52.0
FRUIT COCKTAIL (CANNED, HEAVY SYRUP)	96.0
FRUIT COCKTAIL (CANNED, JUICE)	58.0
FRUIT JELLIES	20000.0
FRUIT PUNCH DRINK (CANNED)	44000.0
FRUITCAKE	21.2
FUDGE, CHOCOLATE, PLAIN	42.0
GELATIN DESSERT	17.0
GINGER ALE	64000.0
GINGERBREAD CAKE	32.3
GOLDEN GRAHAMS CEREAL	24.0
GRAHAM CRACKER (PLAIN)	22.0
GRAPE DRINK (CANNED)	52000.0
GRAPE JUICE (CANNED)	76.0
GRAPE SODA	92000.0
GRAPEFRUIT (CANNED, SYRUP)	78.0
GRAPEFRUIT (RAW)	20.0
GRAPEFRUIT JUICE (SWEETENED)	56.0
GRAPEFRUIT JUICE (UNSWEETENED)	48.0
GRAPE-NUTS CEREAL	15.3
GRAPES (RAW)	1800.0
GROUND BEEF (BROILED, LEAN & FAT)	40.0
GROUND BEEF (BROILED, LEAN)	20.0
GUM DROPS	50000.0
HALF AND HALF (CREAM)	22.9
HAMBURGER	24.7
HARD CANDY	56000.0
HOLLANDAISE (WATER)	45.6
HONEY	558.0
HONEY NUT CHEERIOS CEREAL	15.3
HONEYDEW MELON	24.0
ICE CREAM (VANLLA,11% FAT)	53.4
ICE CREAM (VANLLA,16% FAT)	55.5
ICE MILK (VANILLA, 3%)	49.5
ICE MILK (VANILLA, 4% FAT)	51.3
IMITATION CREAMER (POWDERED)	2020.0
IMITATION SOUR DRESSING	42.8

IMITATION WHIPPED TOPING	2040.0
ITALIAN BREAD	12.8
ITALIAN SALAD DRESSING (LOW CAL)	400.0
ITALIAN SALAD DRESSING (REGULAR)	200.0
JAMS AND FRUIT PRESERVES	20000.0
JELLY BEANS	52000.0
JERUSALEM-ARTICHOKE	13.0
KIWIFRUIT	22.0
LAMB (LEG, LEAN & FAT, ROASTED)	40.0
LAMB (LEG, LEAN, ROASTED)	20.0
LAMB CHOPS (ARM, LEAN & FAT, BRAISED)	40.0
LAMB CHOPS (ARM, LEAN, BRAISED)	20.0
LAMB CHOPS (LOIN, LEAN & FAT, BROIL)	40.0
LAMB CHOPS (LOIN, LEAN, BROIL)	20.0
LAMB RIB (LEAN & FAT, ROASTED)	40.0
LAMB RIB (LEAN, ROASTED)	20.0
LARD	4002.0
LEMON JUICE	32.0
LEMON MERINGUE PIE	20.5
LEMONADE	42000.0
LEMON-LIME SODA	78000.0
LUCKY CHARMS CEREAL	15.3
MACARONI	11.1
MACARONI AND CHEESE	44.7
MALTED MILK (CHOCOLATE)	46.4
MALTED MILK (REGULAR)	44.9
MALT-O-MEAL	33.0
MANGO (RAW)	70.0
MARGARINE (REGULAR, HARD)	22.0
MARGARINE (IMITATION 40% FAT)	22.0
MARGARINE (REGULAR, HARD, 80% FAT)	22.0
MARGARINE (REGULR, SOFT)	22.0
MARGARINE (REGULR, SOFT, 80% FAT)	22.0
MARGARINE (SPREAD, HARD, 60% FAT)	22.0
MARGARINE (SPREAD, SOFT, 60% FAT)	22.0
MARSHMALLOWS	46.0
MAYONNAISE (IMITATION)	4020.0
MAYONNAISE (REGULAR)	42.0

MAYONNAISE SALAD DRESSING	8040.0
MILK (1% LOW FAT)	23.0
MILK (2% LOW FAT)	42.7
MILK (WHOLE)	42.8
MOLASSES	44000.0
MOZZARELLA CHEESE (WHOLE MILK)	40.3
MOZZARELLA CHESE (SKIM MILK)	20.3
MUENSTER CHEESE	40.0
MUSHROOM GRAVY	28.7
NATURE VALLEY GRANOLA CEREAL	12.7
NECTARINES	32.0
OATMEAL & RAISIN COOKIES	24.0
OATMEAL (FLAVORED)	12.4
OATMEAL BREAD	11.2
ONION RINGS	16.0
ONIONS (RAW)	12.0
ORANGE & GRAPEFRUIT JUICE	50.0
ORANGE (RAW)	30.0
ORANGE JUICE (CANNED)	50.0
ORANGE JUICE (FRESH)	26.0
ORANGE SODA	92000.0
PANCAKES (BUCKWHEAT)	12.0
PANCAKES (PLAIN)	16.0
PAPAYA	34.0
PARMESAN CHEESE	40.2
PARMESAN CHEESE	40.2
PARSNIPS	22.5
PEACH PIE	30.1
PEACHES (CANNED, HEAVY SYRUP)	102.0
PEACHES (CANNED, JUICE)	29.0
PEACHES (DRIED)	32.7
PEACHES (FRESH)	20.0
PEANUT BUTTER COOKIE	14.0
PEAR (CANNED, HEAVY SYRUP)	98.0
PEAR (CANNED, JUICE)	64.0
PEAR (FRESH)	37.5
PECAN PIE	20.1
PICKLES (CUCUMBER)	600.0

PICKLES (CUCUMBER, DILL)	200.0
PICKLES (CUCUMBER, SWEET)	1000.0
PIE CRUST	14.1
PINEAPPLE (CANNED, HEAVY SYRUP)	104.0
PINEAPPLE (CANNED, JUICE)	78.0
PINEAPPLE (FRESH)	38.0
PINEAPPLE JUICE (UNSWEETENED)	68.0
PINEAPPLE-GRAPEFRUIT JUICE DRINK	46000.0
PITA BREAD	11.0
PLANTAINS	42.8
PLUMS (CANNED, HEAVY SYRUP)	120.0
PLUMS (CANNED, JUICE)	76.0
PLUMS (FRESH)	18.0
POPCORN (SYRUP)	22.5
POPSICLE	36000.0
PORK (CURED, BACON)	40.0
PORK (CURED, CANADIAN BACON)	40.2
PORK (CURED, HAM, LEAN & FAT)	40.0
PORK (CURED, HAM, LEAN)	40.0
PORK (LINK)	20.0
PORK (LUNCHEON MEAT, CANNED)	40.4
PORK (LUNCHEON MEAT, HAM, LEAN & FAT)	40.4
PORK (LUNCHEON MEAT, HAM, LEAN)	20.2
PORK (ROASTED HAM, LEAN)	20.0
PORK CHOP LOIN (BROILED, LEAN & FAT)	40.0
PORK CHOP LOIN (BROILED, LEAN)	20.0
PORK CHOP LOIN (FRIED, LEAN & FAT)	40.0
PORK CHOP LOIN (FRIED, LEAN)	20.0
PORK FRESH (ROASTED HAM, LEAN & FAT)	40.0
PORK RIBS (ROASTED, LEAN & FAT)	40.0
PORK RIBS (ROASTED, LEAN)	20.0
PORK SHOULDER (BRAISED, LEAN & FAT)	40.0
PORK SHOULDER (BRAISED, LEAN)	20.0
POTATO CHIPS	20.0
POTATO SALAD (MAYONNAISE)	28.0
POTATOES (AU GRATIN)	52.4
POTATOES (BAKED, NO SKIN)	22.7
POTATOES (BAKED, WITH SKIN)	20.4

POTATOES (BOILED)	18.0
POTATOES (FRENCH FRIES, BAKED)	17.0
POTATOES (FRENCH FRIES, FRIED)	20.0
POTATOES (HASHED BROWN)	17.6
POTATOES (MASHED)	16.0
POTATOES (SCALLOPED)	52.4
POUND CAKE	19.8
PRETZELS	13.0
PRODUCT 19 CEREAL	16.0
PROVOLONE CHEESE	40.3
PRUNE JUICE	22.5
PRUNES (DRIED)	31.0
PUMPERNICKEL BREAD	10.6
PUMPKIN (CANNED)	13.3
PUMPKIN (FRESH)	12.0
PUMPKIN PIE	12.7
QUICHE LORRAINE	44.5
RADISHES	200.0
RAISIN BRAN CEREAL	10.5
RAISIN BREAD	13.0
RAISINS	34.5
RASPBERRIES (SWEETENED)	55.5
RELISH (SWEET)	100.0
RHUBARB (SWEETENED)	150.0
RICE (BROWN)	20.0
RICE (WHITE)	25.0
RICE KRISPIES CEREAL	25.0
RICE PUDDING (nonfat milk)	13.5
RICOTTA CHEESE (WHOLE MILK)	40.5
ROAST BEEF SANDWICH	23.1
ROLLS (DINNER)	28.0
ROLLS (FRANKFURTER & HAMBURGER)	13.3
ROLLS (HARD)	12.0
ROLLS (HOAGIE OR SUBMARINE)	13.1
ROOT BEER	84000.0
RYE WAFERS (WHOLE-GRAIN)	15.0
SALAMI (DRY)	40.4
SALAMI (NOT DRY)	40.3

SALTINES	18.0
SANDWICH SPREAD (BEEF & PORK)	44.0
SAUSAGE (BROWN AND SERVE)	40.0
SEAWEED (KELP)	60.0
SELF-RISING FLOUR (UNSIFTED)	15.5
SEMI SWEET CHOCOLATE	47.7
SHEETCAKE (NO FROSTING)	26.3
SHEETCAKE (WHITE FROSTING)	51.3
SHERBET	55.2
SHORTBREAD COOKIE	20.0
SHREDDED WHEAT CEREAL	11.5
SNACK CAKES (DEVIL'S FOOD & CRÈME)	34.0
SNACK CAKES (SPONGE & CRÈME)	54.0
SOLE (BAKED IN MARGARINE)	20.0
SOLE (BAKED IN BUTTER)	40.0
SOUR CREAM	42.9
SPAGHETTI (SOFT)	12.8
SPAGHETTI (TOMATO SAUCE, CHEESE)	13.0
SPINACH SOUFFLE	40.5
SQUASH (WINTER)	18.0
STEAK (BROILED, SIRLOIN)	20.0
STRAWBERRIES (FRESH)	15.0
STRAWBERRIES (FROZEN, SWEETENED)	55.5
SUGAR (BROWN)	424000.0
SUGAR (WHITE)	398000.0
SUGAR COOKIE	31.0
SUGAR SMACKS CEREAL	25.0
SUPER SUGAR CRISP CEREAL	26.0
SWEET POTATOE PIE	58000.0
SWEET POTATOES (BAKED)	21.0
SWEETPOTATOES (CANNED)	12.0
SWEETPOTATOES (CANNED, MASHED)	23.6
SWISS CHEESE	40.3
SWISS CHEESE	40.3
SYRUP (LIGHT, CHOCOLATE FLAVORED)	44.0
SYRUP (CORN, MAPLE)	64000.0
SYRUP (THICK, CHOCOLATE FLAVORED)	21.0
TANGERINE JUICE	60.0

TANGERINES (CANNED, LIGHT SYRUP)	82.0
TANGERINES (FRESH)	18.0
TAPIOCA PUDDING (nonfat milk)	18.7
TARTAR SAUCE	240.0
THOUSAND ISLAND DRESSING	440.0
TOASTER PASTRIES	38.0
TOMATO & VEGETABLE SOUP	12.0
TOMATO PASTE	10.9
TOMATO PUREE	12.5
TOMATO SOUP (WATER)	17.0
TOTAL CEREAL	14.7
TRIX CEREAL	25.0
TUNA SALAD (Imitation mayonnaise)	21.2
TURKEY (LIGHT & DARK, ROASTED)	20.0
TURKEY (ROASTED)	20.0
TURKEY AND GRAVY	22.0
TURKEY HAM (CURED)	40.0
TURKEY LOAF	20.0
TURKEY PATTIES (BATTERED, FRIED)	22.2
TURNIPS	16.0
VANILLA PUDDING (nonfat milk)	33.0
VANILLA SHAKE	49.1
VANILLA WAFERS	29.0
VEAL CUTLET (BROILED, ROASTED, BRAISED)	20.0
VEAL RIB (BROILED, ROASTED, BRAISED)	20.0
VEGETABLE & BEEF SOUP	22.5
VIENNA BREAD	13.0
VIENNA SAUSAGE	40.0
WATER CHESTNUTS	34.0
WATERMELON	23.3
WHEAT BREAD	10.1
WHEAT FLOUR (ALL-PURPOSE, SIFTED	14.7
WHEAT FLOUR (ALL-PURPOSE, UNSIFTED)	14.6
WHEATIES CEREAL	15.3
WHITE BREAD	12.0
WHITE BREAD CRUMBS	11.0
WHITE BREAD CUBES	15.0
WHITE CAKE (WHITE FROSTING)	31.2

YELLOW CAKE (CHOCOLATE FROSTING)	29.0
YOGURT (FRUIT, LOW FAT MILK)	48.6
YOGURT (PLAIN, LOW FAT MILK)	42.7
YOGURT (WHOLE MILK)	42.8

EAT FOODS FROM THIS TABLE FOR ONE WEEK THEN SWITCH TO 'GREEN' TABLE ONE (DURING WEIGHT LOSS PHASE)

The Plateau-proof Turbo 'Green' Rotation Two Table (FP values)

ALFALFA SEEDS (SPROUTED, RAW)	0.0
ALL-BRAN CEREAL	1.1
APPLES (DRIED, SULFURED)	0.0
APRICOTS (DRIED)	0.0
APRICOTS (RAW)	0.0
ARTICHOKES (GLOBE, COOKED)	0.0
ASPARAGUS (CANNED)	0.0
ASPARAGUS (FROZEN)	0.0
BARLEY (PEARLED, LIGHT)	0.6
BEAN SPROUTS	0.0
BEET GREENS	0.0
BEETS (CANNED)	0.0
BEETS (COOKED, DRAINED)	0.0
BLACK BEANS (COOKED, DRAINED)	0.3
BLACK-EYED PEAS, DRY, COOKED	0.4
BRAN FLAKES (40%)	0.0
BROCCOLI (FROZEN, COOKED, DRAINED)	0.0
BROCCOLI (RAW, COOKED, DRAINED)	0.0
BRUSSELS SPROUTS	0.8
BUCKWHEAT FLOUR (LIGHT, SIFTED)	0.8
BULGUR	0.8
CABBAGE (CHINESE)	0.0
CABBAGE (COMMON)	0.0
CABBAGE (RED)	0.0
CABBAGE (SAVOY)	0.0
CAROB FLOUR	0.0
CARROTS (FROZEN, COOKED)	0.0
CARROTS (RAW)	0.0
CAULIFLOWER	0.0
CELERY (PASCAL, RAW)	0.0
CHERRIES (SOUR, CANNED, WATER)	0.0

CHICKPEAS	1.3
CLAMS	0.4
COD	0.6
COLLARDS	0.0
CORN (CREAM, CANNED)	1.1
CORN (RAW, WHITE)	1.5
CORN GRITS (WHITE)	0.0
CORN GRITS (YELLOW)	0.0
CRABMEAT	0.6
CRACKED-WHEAT BREAD	1.9
DAB	1.0
DATES	1.1
EGG NOODLES	1.3
EGGPLANT	0.0
EGGS (WHITE, RAW)	0.0
ENDIVE	0.0
EVAPORATED MILK (NONFAT)	0.2
FIGS (DRIED)	1.5
FLOUNDER	0.3
FLOUNDER (BAKED IN VEG OIL)	1.7
FLOUNDER (BAKED, NO FAT)	0.3
GRAPEFRUIT (RAW)	0.0
GREAT NORTHERN BEANS (DRY, DRAINED)	0.3
GREEN PEAS (SOUP)	1.7
GURNARD	1.8
HADDOCK	0.4
HAKE	0.8
HAKE (S. AFRICAN)	0.9
HONEYDEW MELON	0.0
JERUSALEM-ARTICHOKE	0.0
KALE	1.1
KING CRAB (WHITE MEAT)	0.2
KIWIFRUIT	0.0
KOHLRABI	0.0
LEMON SOLE	1.4
LEMONS (RAW)	0.0
LENTILS	0.3
LETTUCE (BUTTER-HEAD)	0.0

LETTUCE (CRISP-HEAD)	0.9
LETTUCE (LOOSE LEAF)	0.0
LIMA BEANS	0.3
MACARONI	0.6
MACKEREL	0.3
MILK (NONFAT)	0.5
MUSHROOMS (CANNED)	0.0
MUSHROOMS (RAW)	0.0
MUSTARD GREENS	0.0
NONFAT DRY MILK	0.1
NORWAY LOBSTER (WHITE MEAT)	0.3
OATMEAL (FLAVORED)	1.8
OKRA	0.0
ONION SOUP	0.0
ONIONS (RAW)	0.0
ONIONS (RAW, SPRING)	0.0
ORANGE (RAW)	0.0
OYSTERS (RAW)	1.0
PAPAYA	0.0
PARSNIPS	0.0
PEA BEANS (DRY)	0.3
PEACHES (DRIED)	0.8
PEACHES (FRESH)	0.0
PEAS (CANNED, GREEN)	0.6
PEAS (FRESH, GREEN)	0.1
PEAS (POD)	0.0
PEPPERS (HOT GREEN CHILI)	0.0
PEPPERS (HOT RED CHILI)	0.0
PEPPERS (SWEET GREEN)	0.0
PEPPERS (SWEET RED)	0.0
PILCHARD	0.9
PINTO BEANS	0.3
PLANTAINS (GREEN)	0.0
PLUMS (FRESH)	0.0
POTATOES (BAKED, NO SKIN)	0.0
POTATOES (BAKED, WITH SKIN)	0.0
POTATOES (BOILED)	0.0
PRAWN	1.4

PRUNES (DRIED)	0.0
PUMPKIN (CANNED)	1.5
PUMPKIN (FRESH)	0.0
RAISINS	0.9
RED KIDNEY BEANS	0.3
REDFISH	0.8
REFRIED BEANS	0.8
RICE (BROWN)	0.9
SALMON	0.5
SALMON (CANNED)	1.3
SALMON (RED, BAKED)	1.1
SAUERKRAUT	0.0
SCALLOP	0.9
SEAWEED (SPIRULINA)	0.6
SHRIMP	1.4
SHRIMP	0.2
SKATE RAY	1.7
SNAP BEAN (GREEN)	0.0
SNAP BEAN (YELLOW)	0.0
SOLE	1.0
SOLE (BAKED IN VEG OIL)	1.7
SOLE (BAKED, NO FAT)	0.3
SOY SAUCE	0.0
SPAGHETTI (FIRM)	0.6
SPAGHETTI (SOFT)	0.9
SPINACH (CANNED)	0.8
SPINACH (FRESH)	0.0
SPINACH (FROZEN)	0.0
SQUID	1.4
SWEET POTATOES (BAKED)	0.0
SWEETPOTATOES (CANNED)	0.0
SWEETPOTATOES (CANNED, MASHED)	0.9
TANGERINES (FRESH)	0.0
TOMATO PASTE	1.0
TOMATOES (FRESH)	0.0
TUNA (CANNED, LIGHT, VEG OIL, DRAINNED)	1.4
TUNA (CANNED, LIGHT, WATER)	0.2
TURNIP GREENS (FRESH)	0.0

TURNIP GREENS (FROZEN)	0.9
TURNIPS	0.0
VEGETABLE JUICE	0.0
VEGETABLES (MIXED)	0.0
WATER CHESTNUTS	0.0
WHEAT FLOUR (ALL-PURPOSE, SIFTED	0.4
WHEAT FLOUR (ALL-PURPOSE, UNSIFTED)	0.3
WHOLE-WHEAT FLOUR	0.6
YOGURT (NONFAT MILK)	0.0

EAT FOODS FROM THIS TABLE AND FROM GREEN TABLE TWO FOR ONE WEEK THEN SWITCH TO 'YELLOW' TABLE ONE (DURING WEIGHT MAINTENANCE PHASE). ALSO CHOOSE ISOLATED ITEMS FROM THIS TABLE TO MAKE A BALANCED DIET WITH ANY ITEMS IN 'GREEN' TABLE TWO.

The Plateau-proof Turbo 'Yellow' Rotation Two Table (FP values)

APPLES (RAW, UNPEELED)	4.5
APPLESAUCE (CANNED,UNSWEETENED)	4.5
APRICOT (CANNED, HEAVY SYRUP)	2.5
APRICOT NECTAR	2.5
APRICOTS (CANNED, IN JUICE)	2.5
BAGELS (EGG)	3.8
BAGELS (PLAIN)	3.8
BAMBOO SHOOTS (CANNED)	2.3
BANANAS	4.5
BASS	2.7
BEER (LIGHT)	2.5
BEER (REGULAR)	2.5
BLACKBERRIES (RAW)	4.5
BLUE WHITING	2.9
BLUEBERRIES (RAW)	4.5
BOSTON BROWN BREAD	2.3
BOUILLON (DEHYDRATED)	4.5
BREADCRUMBS	4.3
BRILL	2.7
CANTALOUP	2.3
CARP	2.3
CATFISH	3.3
CATSUP	3.4
CELERY SEED	4.5
CHERRIES (RAW, SWEET)	4.5
CHESTNUTS (ROASTED)	2.7
CLAM CHOWDER (MANHATTAN, NO MILK)	2.3
CLUB SODA	4.5

COCKLE	3.4
COCOA POWDER (NONFAT DRY MILK)	4.0
COFFEE	4.5
COLA (DIET)	4.5
CORN (RAW, YELLOW)	2.3
CORNMEAL	2.0
CRACKED-WHEAT BREAD	2.3
CRANBERRY JUICE COCKTAL	4.5
CUCUMBER (WITH PEEL)	4.5
DANDELION GREENS	2.3
ENGLISH MUFFINS (PLAIN)	3.4
FISH STICKS	2.3
FRENCH BREAD	4.6
FRUIT COCKTAIL (CANNED, JUICE)	2.5
GRAPE JUICE (CANNED)	2.5
GRAPEFRUIT JUICE (UNSWEETENED)	2.5
GRAPES (RAW)	4.5
GREY MULLET	4.2
HADDOCK (BREADED, FRIED)	2.6
ITALIAN BREAD	3.0
ITALIAN SALAD DRESSING (LOW CAL)	4.5
LEMON JUICE	4.5
LING	2.4
LIQUOR (GIN, RUM, VODKA, WHISKY, COGNAC...)	4.5
LOBSTER (BROWN MEAT)	2.5
MANGO (RAW)	4.5
MELBA TOAST	2.5
MINESTRONE SOUP	3.4
MISO	2.2
MIXED GRAIN BREAD	4.3
MUSSEL	2.1
MUSTARD (YELLOW)	4.5
NECTARINES	4.5
NORWAY POUT	2.8
OATMEAL (PLAIN)	2.3
OATMEAL BREAD	2.5
ORANGE & GRAPEFRUIT JUICE	2.5
ORANGE JUICE (CANNED, UNSWEETENED)	2.5

ORANGE JUICE (FRESH, UNSWEETENED)	2.5
OYSTER	2.3
PANCAKES (BUCKWHEAT)	4.5
PEACHES (CANNED, JUICE)	2.5
PEAR (CANNED, JUICE)	2.5
PEAR (FRESH)	4.5
PICKLES (CUCUMBER)	4.5
PICKLES (CUCUMBER, DILL)	4.5
PINEAPPLE (CANNED, JUICE)	2.5
PINEAPPLE (FRESH)	4.5
PINEAPPLE JUICE (UNSWEETENED)	2.5
PITA BREAD	3.3
PLUMS (CANNED, JUICE)	2.5
POLLACK	2.7
POPCORN (AIR-POPPED)	2.5
PRETZELS	4.8
PRUNE JUICE	2.5
PUMPERNICKEL BREAD	4.4
RADISHES	4.5
RAISIN BRAN CEREAL	4.0
RAISIN BREAD	4.8
RICE (WHITE)	2.5
ROLLS (HARD)	4.3
RYE BREAD (LIGHT)	2.2
RYE WAFERS (WHOLE-GRAIN)	4.5
SALMON (SMOKED)	4.5
SALTINES	4.5
SARDINES (CANNED, VEG OIL, ATLANTIC)	2.2
SCALLOPS (BREADED)	3.2
SEAWEED (KELP)	4.5
SELF-RISING FLOUR (UNSIFTED)	2.9
SHREDDED WHEAT CEREAL	4.0
SHRIMP (FRIED VEG OIL, NOT BREADED / BATTERED)	3.0
SOYBEANS	2.4
SPECIAL K CEREAL (LOW CARB)	2.5
SPRAT	2.0
SQUASH (SUMMER)	2.3
SQUASH (WINTER)	2.3

STRAWBERRIES (FRESH)	4.5
TANGERINE JUICE	2.5
TANGERINES (CANNED, LIGHT SYRUP)	2.5
TEA (BREWED, UNSWEETENED)	4.5
TOFU	2.5
TOMATO & VEGETABLE SOUP	4.5
TOMATO JUICE	2.5
TOMATO PUREE	2.5
TOMATO SOUP (WATER)	4.5
TOMATOES (CANNED)	2.3
TORTILLAS (CORN)	2.3
TROUT	4.6
VEGETARIAN SOUP	4.5
VIENNA BREAD	4.8
WATERMELON	3.0
WHEAT BREAD	2.2
WHEAT CRACKERS	4.5

AVOID THE FOODS IN THIS TABLE DURING THIS ROTATION

The Plateau-proof Turbo 'Red' Rotation Two Table (FP values)

ALMONDS (SLIVERED)	11.8
AMERICAN CHEESE	58.6
AMERICAN CHEESE SPREAD	54.2
ANGELFOOD CAKE	5.2
ANGLER	7.8
APPLE JUICE (CANNED)	7.0
APPLE PIE	30.9
APPLE PIE (FRIED)	41.7
APPLESAUCE (CANNED, SWEETENED)	9.5
AVOCADOS (CALIFORNIA)	33.9
AVOCADOS (FLORIDA)	24.5
BARBECUE SAUCE	7.0
BEAN WITH BACON SOUP	43.5
BEANS (CANNED, FRANKFURTER)	49.8
BEANS (PORK, SWEET SAUCE)	47.2
BEANS (PORK, TOMATO SAUCE)	44.5
BEEF (DRIED)	23.3
BEEF (LEAN & FAT CHUCK BLADE)	31.3
BEEF (LEAN & FAT, BOTTOM ROUND)	26.5
BEEF (LEAN, BOTTOM ROUND)	24.1
BEEF (LEAN, CHUCK BLADE)	26.9
BEEF AND VEGETABLE STEW	27.6
BEEF BROTH (BOULLION)	21.5
BEEF GRAVY	27.7
BEEF HEART (BRAISED)	21.0
BEEF LIVER (FRIED)	24.1
BEEF NOODLE SOUP	22.7
BEEF POTPIE	29.4
BEEF ROAST (LEAN, EYE O RND)	21.2
BEEF ROAST (LEAN & FAT, EYE O RND)	27.1
BEEF ROAST (LEAN & FAT, RIBS)	32.2
BEEF ROAST (LEAN, RIBS)	26.5

BEEF STEAK (LEAN, SIRLOIN, BROIL)	24.8
BISCUIT BAKING MIX	9.3
BLUE CHEESE	57.6
BLUE CHEESE SALAD DRESSING	76.1
BLUEBERRIES (FROZEN, SWEETENED)	5.0
BLUEBERRY MUFFINS	10.1
BLUEBERRY PIE	28.2
BOLOGNA	55.0
BRAN MUFFINS	6.1
BRAUNSCHWEIGER	54.2
BRAZIL NUTS	21.6
BREAD STUFFING (DRY MIX)	15.7
BROWN GRAVY (DRY MIX)	23.0
BROWNIES WITH NUTS	32.1
BUTTER	469.6
BUTTERMILK (DRIED)	49.7
BUTTERMILK (LIQUID)	41.5
CAKE & PASTRY FLOUR	5.6
CAMEMBERT CHEESE	56.5
CANDY (MILK CHOCOLATE, ALMONDS)	66.1
CANDY (MILK CHOCOLATE, PEANUTS)	61.5
CANDY (MILK CHOCOLATE, PLAIN)	74.9
CANDY (MILK CHOCOLATE, RICE CRISPIES)	70.2
CAP'N CRUNCH CEREAL	16.5
CARAMEL	20.2
CARROT CAKE (CREME CHESE FROSTING)	30.9
CASHEW NUTS (DRY ROASTD)	14.8
CASHEW NUTS (ROASTED, OIL)	13.7
CEREAL (100% NATURAL)	19.7
CHEDDAR CHEESE	58.3
CHEERIOS CEREAL	7.3
CHEESE CRACKERS (PEANUT SANDWICH)	51.5
CHEESE CRACKERS (PLAIN)	47.0
CHEESE SAUCE WITH MILK	54.3
CHEESEBURGER	54.2
CHEESECAKE	74.7
CHERRY PIE	27.7
CHERRY PIE (FRIED)	41.7

CHICKEN (CANNED)	41.8
CHICKEN (LIGHT & DARK, STEWED)	21.3
CHICKEN A LA KING	31.3
CHICKEN AND NOODLES	26.6
CHICKEN BREAST (FRIED, BATTERED)	27.6
CHICKEN BREAST (FRIED, FLOUR)	24.0
CHICKEN BREAST (ROASTED)	20.5
CHICKEN CHOW MEIN	20.0
CHICKEN DRUMSTICK (FRIED, BATTERED)	28.0
CHICKEN DRUMSTICK (ROASTED)	20.8
CHICKEN DRUMSTICK, (FRIED, FLOUR)	25.1
CHICKEN FRANKFURTER	47.0
CHICKEN GRAVY (CANNED)	32.8
CHICKEN GRAVY (DRY MIX)	23.0
CHICKEN LIVER	20.9
CHICKEN NOODLE SOUP	22.3
CHICKEN POTPIE	33.1
CHICKEN RICE SOUP	22.3
CHICKEN ROLL	24.3
CHILI	8.1
CHOCOLATE (SWEET, DARK)	99.6
CHOCOLATE (FOR BAKING, BITTER)	33.9
CHOCOLATE CHIP COOKIES	28.0
CHOCOLATE MILK (LOWFAT 1%)	46.9
CHOCOLATE MILK (LOWFAT 2%)	55.0
CHOCOLATE MILK (REGULAR)	60.7
CHOCOLATE PUDDING	54.3
CHOCOLATE SHAKE	58.5
CHOP SUEY (BEEF & PORK)	25.5
CHOW MEIN NOODLES	8.4
CLAM CHOWDER (NEW ENGLAND, MILK)	47.5
COCOA POWDER (REGULAR)	54.1
COCONUT (RAW)	115.2
COCONUT (SHREDDED, DRIED, SWEETENED)	114.7
COFFEE CREAM (LIGHT)	89.8
COFFEECAKE (CRUMB)	15.4
COLA (REGULAR)	9.5
CONDENSED MILK (SWEETENED)	64.2

CONGER	6.5
CORN CHIPS	20.3
CORN FLAKES	5.0
CORN MUFFINS	7.6
CORN OIL	981000.1
CORNED BEEF (CANNED)	46.7
COTTAGE CHEESE (FRUIT)	51.2
COTTAGE CHEESE (LARGE CURDS, CREAMED)	53.3
COTTAGE CHEESE (LOWFAT 2%)	48.8
COTTAGE CHEESE (UNCREAMED)	40.2
CRAB (BROWN MEAT)	7.2
CRAB (WHITE MEAT)	9.0
CRACKERS (SNACK)	4502.5
CRANBERRY SAUCE (SWEATENED, CANNED)	5.0
CREAM CHEESE	73.3
CREAM OF CHICKEN SOUP (MILK)	52.0
CREAM OF CHICKEN SOUP (WATER)	30.7
CREAM OF MUSHROM SOUP (MILK)	54.6
CREAM OF MUSHROOM SOUP (WATER)	20.4
CREAM OF WHEAT	5.0
CREME PIE	54.2
CROISSANTS	15.9
CUSTARD (BAKED)	14.0
CUSTARD PIE	16.0
DANISH PASTRY (FRUIT)	22.5
DANISH PASTRY (PLAIN)	24.3
DEVIL'S FOOD CAKE (CHOCOLATE FROSTING)	25.3
DOGFISH	5.2
DOUGHNUTS (CAKE TYPE, PLAIN)	23.2
DOUGHNUTS (YEAST-LEAVENED, GLAZED)	29.3
DUCK (ROASTED)	27.2
EEL	22.7
EGG NOG	21.3
EGGS (FRIED)	5.4
EGGS (YOLK, RAW)	7.6
ENCHILADA	10.8
ENG MUFFIN (BACON, EGG, CHEESE)	53.4
EVAPORATED MILK (WHOLE)	57.6

FETA CHEESE	58.2
FIG BARS	11.5
FILBERTS (HAZELNUTS)	21.7
FISH SANDWICH (CHEESE)	52.0
FISH SANDWICH (NO CHEESE)	11.7
FLOUNDER (BAKED IN BUTTER)	47.5
FRANKFURTER	55.8
FRENCH SALAD DRESSING (LOW CAL)	9005.0
FRENCH SALAD DRESSING (REGULAR)	40505.0
FRENCH TOAST	7.8
FROOT LOOPS CEREAL	7.3
FROSTED FLAKES CEREAL	5.0
FRUIT COCKTAIL (CANNED, HEAVY SYRUP)	5.0
FRUIT JELLIES	9.5
FRUIT PUNCH DRINK (CANNED)	9.5
FRUITCAKE	21.5
FUDGE, CHOCOLATE, PLAIN	25.5
GELATIN DESSERT	5.0
GINGER ALE	9.5
GINGERBREAD CAKE	15.1
GOLDEN GRAHAMS CEREAL	7.3
GRAHAM CRACKER (PLAIN)	7.0
GRAPE DRINK (CANNED)	9.5
GRAPE SODA	9.5
GRAPEFRUIT (CANNED, SYRUP)	5.0
GRAPEFRUIT JUICE (SWEETENED)	5.0
GRAPE-NUTS CEREAL	5.0
GROUND BEEF (BROILED, LEAN & FAT)	29.0
GROUND BEEF (BROILED, LEAN)	28.2
GUM DROPS	9.5
HALF AND HALF (CREAM)	71.9
HALIBUT	5.5
HALIBUT (BROILED, BUTTER & LEMON JUICE)	7.6
HAMBURGER	31.1
HARD CANDY	9.5
HERRING	12.4
HERRING (PICKLED)	6.8
HOLLANDAISE (WATER)	69.3

HONEY	5.0
HONEY NUT CHEERIOS CEREAL	6.5
ICE CREAM (VANLLA,11% FAT)	74.3
ICE CREAM (VANLLA,16% FAT)	87.0
ICE MILK (VANILLA, 3%)	53.9
ICE MILK (VANILLA, 4% FAT)	65.0
IMITATION CREAMER (POWDERED)	4540.0
IMITATION SOUR DRESSING	96.2
IMITATION WHIPPED TOPING	3640.0
ITALIAN SALAD DRESSING (REGULAR)	40500.0
JAMS AND FRUIT PRESERVES	7.0
JELLY BEANS	9.5
JOHN DORY	14.6
LAMB (LEG, LEAN & FAT, ROASTED)	28.2
LAMB (LEG, LEAN, ROASTED)	24.4
LAMB CHOPS (ARM, LEAN & FAT, BRAISED)	29.9
LAMB CHOPS (ARM, LEAN, BRAISED)	25.7
LAMB CHOPS (LOIN, LEAN & FAT, BROIL)	29.8
LAMB CHOPS (LOIN, LEAN, BROIL)	25.0
LAMB RIB (LEAN & FAT, ROASTED)	33.9
LAMB RIB (LEAN, ROASTED)	26.7
LARD	922546.3
LEMON MERINGUE PIE	16.6
LEMONADE	9.5
LEMON-LIME SODA	9.5
LOBSTER (WHITE MEAT)	16.8
LUCKY CHARMS CEREAL	6.5
MACADAMIA NUTS (OIL ROASTED)	46.5
MACARONI AND CHEESE	52.5
MALTED MILK (CHOCOLATE)	59.5
MALTED MILK (REGULAR)	59.1
MALT-O-MEAL	45.0
MARGARINE (REGULAR, HARD)	49500.1
MARGARINE (IMITATION 40% FAT)	396.2
MARGARINE (REGULAR, HARD, 80% FAT)	409.7
MARGARINE (REGULR, SOFT)	49500.1
MARGARINE (REGULR, SOFT, 80% FAT)	823.7
MARGARINE (SPREAD, HARD, 60% FAT)	313.3

MARGARINE (SPREAD, SOFT, 60% FAT)	623.6
MARSHMALLOWS	5.0
MAYONNAISE (IMITATION)	13540.0
MAYONNAISE (REGULAR)	49540.1
MAYONNAISE SALAD DRESSING	22540.0
MEGRIM	13.5
MILK (1% LOW FAT)	44.4
MILK (2% LOW FAT)	48.6
MILK (WHOLE)	55.0
MIXED NUTS (DRY ROASTED, NO HONEY)	16.9
MIXED NUTS (OIL ROASTED, NO HONEY)	14.5
MOLASSES	9.5
MOZZARELLA CHEESE (WHOLE MILK)	52.7
MOZZARELLA CHESE (NONFAT MILK)	10.0
MUENSTER CHEESE	55.4
MUSHROOM GRAVY	29.0
NATURE VALLEY GRANOLA CEREAL	21.0
OATMEAL & RAISIN COOKIES	20.2
OCEAN PERCH (FRIED, BREADED)	5.8
OLIVE OIL	972000.2
OLIVES (BLACK)	9000.0
OLIVES (GREEN)	9000.0
ONION RINGS	25.2
ORANGE SODA	9.5
OYSTERS (FRIED, BREADED)	7.1
PANCAKES (PLAIN)	7.0
PARMESAN CHEESE	58.4
PARMESAN CHEESE	53.3
PEACH PIE	26.9
PEACHES (CANNED, HEAVY SYRUP)	5.0
PEANUT BUTTER	7.3
PEANUT BUTTER COOKIE	23.5
PEANUT OIL	972000.2
PEANUTS (OIL-ROASTED)	7.9
PEAR (CANNED, HEAVY SYRUP)	5.0
PECAN PIE	27.7
PECANS (HALVES)	41.1
PERCH	5.3

PICKLES (CUCUMBER, SWEET)	9.5
PIE CRUST	26.4
PILCHARD (S. AFRICAN)	10.9
PINE NUTS	38.4
PINEAPPLE (CANNED, HEAVY SYRUP)	5.0
PINEAPPLE-GRAPEFRUIT JUICE DRINK	9.5
PISTACHIO NUTS	10.6
PIZZA (CHEESE)	50.7
PLAICE	9.5
PLUMS (CANNED, HEAVY SYRUP)	5.0
POPCORN (SYRUP)	7.3
POPCORN (VEGETABLE OIL)	16.0
POPSICLE	9.5
PORK (CURED, BACON)	30.2
PORK (CURED, CANADIAN BACON)	21.7
PORK (CURED, HAM, LEAN & FAT)	27.8
PORK (CURED, HAM, LEAN)	21.1
PORK (LINK)	26.1
PORK (LUNCHEON MEAT, CANNED)	35.4
PORK (LUNCHEON MEAT, HAM, LEAN & FAT)	22.9
PORK (LUNCHEON MEAT, HAM, LEAN)	21.2
PORK (ROASTED HAM, LEAN)	24.5
PORK CHOP LOIN (BROILED, LEAN & FAT)	28.3
PORK CHOP LOIN (BROILED, LEAN)	24.1
PORK CHOP LOIN (FRIED, LEAN & FAT)	30.6
PORK CHOP LOIN (FRIED, LEAN)	26.1
PORK FRESH (ROASTED HAM, LEAN & FAT)	28.4
PORK RIBS (ROASTED, LEAN & FAT)	28.8
PORK RIBS (ROASTED, LEAN)	25.5
PORK SHOULDER (BRAISED, LEAN & FAT)	28.9
PORK SHOULDER (BRAISED, LEAN)	24.5
POTATO CHIPS	31.6
POTATO SALAD (MAYONNAISE)	53.6
POTATOES (AU GRATIN)	60.3
POTATOES (FRENCH FRIES, BAKED)	12.8
POTATOES (FRENCH FRIES, FRIED)	18.2
POTATOES (HASHED BROWN)	21.2
POTATOES (MASHED)	24.2

POTATOES (SCALLOPED)	59.9
POUND CAKE	33.2
PRODUCT 19 CEREAL	5.0
PROVOLONE CHEESE	54.1
PUMPKIN AND SQUASH KERNELS	8.5
PUMPKIN PIE	23.8
QUICHE LORRAINE	67.7
RASPBERRIES (SWEETENED)	5.0
RED MULLET	6.2
RELISH (SWEET)	9.5
RHUBARB (SWEETENED)	5.0
RICE KRISPIES CEREAL	5.0
RICE PUDDING	54.3
RICOTTA CHEESE (NONFAT MILK)	17.2
RICOTTA CHEESE (WHOLE MILK)	60.5
ROAST BEEF SANDWICH	27.6
ROLLS (FOR FRANKFURTER & HAMBURGER)	5.5
ROLLS (DINNER)	11.5
ROLLS (FOR HOAGIE OR SUBMARINE)	5.9
ROOT BEER	9.5
SAFFLOWER OIL	981000.1
SAITHE	5.5
SALAMI (DRY)	48.8
SALAMI (NOT DRY)	51.1
SALMON (PACIFIC)	74.2
SAND EEL	7.2
SANDWICH SPREAD (BEEF & PORK)	33.5
SAUSAGE (BROWN AND SERVE)	51.4
SEA BREAM	7.5
SEMI SWEET CHOCOLATE	97.8
SESAME SEEDS	9.0
SHEETCAKE (NO FROSTING)	23.3
SHEETCAKE (WHITE FROSTING)	29.5
SHERBET	67.0
SHORTBREAD COOKIE	199.5
SNACK CAKES (DEVIL'S FOOD & CRÈME)	25.1
SNACK CAKES (SPONGE & CRÈME)	31.0
SOLE (BAKED IN BUTTER)	47.5

SOUR CREAM	86.2
SOYBEAN OIL (HYDROGENATED)	981000.2
SOYBEAN-COTTONSEED OIL (HYDROGENATED)	981000.2
SPAGHETTI (MEATBALLS, TOMATO SAUCE)	23.9
SPAGHETTI (TOMATO SAUCE, CHEESE)	41.5
SPINACH SOUFFLE	52.5
STEAK (BROILED, SIRLOIN)	28.5
STRAWBERRIES (FROZEN, SWEETENED)	9.5
SUGAR (BROWN)	9.5
SUGAR (WHITE)	9.5
SUGAR COOKIE	32.1
SUGAR SMACKS CEREAL	7.3
SUNFLOWER OIL	981000.1
SUNFLOWER SEEDS	10.5
SUPER SUGAR CRISP CEREAL	5.0
SWEET POTATOE PIE	13505.2
SWISS CHEESE	54.5
SWISS CHEESE	54.5
SYRUP (LIGHT, CHOCOLATE FLAVORED)	5.0
SYRUP (CORN, MAPLE)	9.5
SYRUP (THICK, CHOCOLATE FLAVORED)	23.5
TACO	9.4
TAHINI	12.0
TAPIOCA PUDDING	84.2
TARTAR SAUCE	36000.0
THOUSAND ISLAND DRESSING	27000.0
TOASTER PASTRIES	18.6
TOMATO SOUP (MILK)	49.1
TOTAL CEREAL	6.5
TRIX CEREAL	5.0
TROUT (BROILED, BUTTER)	47.2
TUNA	9.8
TUNA SALAD	42.7
TURBOT	14.4
TURKEY (LIGHT & DARK, ROASTED)	21.0
TURKEY (ROASTED)	20.5
TURKEY AND GRAVY	22.6
TURKEY HAM (CURED)	21.2

TURKEY LOAF	20.5
TURKEY PATTIES (BATTERED, FRIED)	28.0
TUSK	6.5
VANILLA PUDDING	124.2
VANILLA SHAKE	57.8
VANILLA WAFERS	20.9
VEAL CUTLET (BROILED, ROASTED, BRAISED)	27.1
VEAL RIB (BROILED, ROASTED, BRAISED)	28.3
VEGETABLE & BEEF SOUP	21.5
VIENNA SAUSAGE	49.1
VINEGAR AND OIL SALAD DRESSING	36000.1
WAFFLES	10.3
WALNUTS (BLACK)	10.3
WALNUTS (ENGLISH)	19.7
WHEATIES CEREAL	5.0
WHIPPED TOPPING	87.1
WHIPPING CREAM (HEAVY)	139.9
WHIPPING CREAM (LIGHT)	127.3
WHITE BREAD	10.6
WHITE BREAD CRUMBS	7.3
WHITE BREAD CUBES	7.3
WHITE CAKE (WHITE FROSTING)	23.3
WHITE SAUCE (MILK)	53.0
WHOLE-WHEAT BREAD	5.3
WHOLE-WHEAT WAFERS	9.0
YELLOW CAKE (CHOCOLATE FROSTING)	63.8
YOGURT (FRUIT, LOW FAT MILK)	45.2
YOGURT (PLAIN, LOW FAT MILK)	46.3
YOGURT (WHOLE MILK)	55.8

Chapter Six

Weight Loss Dieting in Hypertension – Facts and Fiction

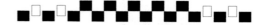

A few years ago while scanning through the hundreds of weight loss products available in the market, I found a company that sold weight loss sunglasses. As ridiculous as that may sound, the only reason that this company was (is) still in business is because some people actually bought the sunglasses. It is difficult to lose weight and to keep it off, so a good number of obese and overweight people get frustrated eventually. The weight loss frustrations have led many to look for the "magic bullet". Unfortunately there is no weight loss "magic bullet". Obesity can only be treated by a lifestyle change that has proper dieting at its core. There are however things that can be done to facilitate weight loss and the maintenance of the new trim look. This chapter takes a brief look at some of the popular and not so popular dieting and weight loss misconceptions and facts.

■

Can dietary supplements affect weight loss?

The answer to this question is a simple NO, at least at this particular time[246-248]. There are two types of dietary supplements:

(1) Vitamins and minerals. Vitamins and minerals are required for the body to function properly. Vitamins and minerals by themselves do not cause weight loss. When a person's diet is not balanced, as may be the case with some restrictive weight loss diets, it is necessary to supplement the diet with vitamins and minerals. Generally, it is sufficient to take a single multivitamin a day. The multivitamins typically have the minerals that your body needs. It is a good idea to ask your pharmacist for recommendations as vitamin pills from certain manufacturers do not dissolve in the gut and end up in the toilet.

(2) Weight loss pills (diet pills). There are more than a hundred diet pills in the market today. A few have a little logic behind them, but most are completely baseless. There is not a single diet pill that meets the standards for use as a weight loss supplement. The Food and Drug Administration (FDA) is responsible for regulating drugs in the United States. These diet pills are technically not considered to be drugs; hence they are not regulated by the FDA. As a result of no regulation, there are an increasing number of ridiculous herbs and portions in the weight loss market. For example, popular diet pills containing ingredients such as ephedra, chromium, chitosan, guar gum, linoleic acid, ginseng, glucomannan, pyruvate, St. John's wort, psyllium, L-carnitine, green tea, hydroxycitric acid, etc, may be good for something, but certainly not for the treatment of obesity. Not one out of the more than hundred diet pills in the market have been proven to cause weight loss. Some of these pills have been shown to be extremely hazardous to health. Before a drug is approved by the

FDA, it is required to pass certain requirements for toxicity (to ensure that it is not going to poison those who will use it). Since the FDA does not regulate the diet supplement industry, manufacturers of diet pills bypass toxicity screening. As a result of this unfortunate practice, many lives are in danger from these diet pills. Let us consider the case of ephedra (ma huang) for example. Ephedra has been marketed as diet pills for several years, until it was recently banned by the FDA. There is evidence that ephedra increases heart rate, blood pressure and resting energy expenditure. The increase in resting energy expenditure is however insignificant in the context of weight loss. There is a lot of evidence that ephedra is extremely hazardous for health[249-257]. It has been shown to cause many health problems, including; severe poisoning of the liver, rhabdomyolysis (destruction of muscles), mania, kidney disease, psychosis, severe depression, agitation, hallucinations, sleep disturbance, suicidal ideation, severe heart disease, and death. The diet pill manufacturers simply replaced ephedra with synephrine (an ephedra-like compound). Synephrine is also now starting to show equally grave health problems[249]. To get more information and updates on ephedra and other diet pills, check the FDA website (www.cfsan.fda.gov).

Does decreasing the amount of iron in the diet affect weight loss?

There is a link between iron metabolism and hypertension (via type II diabetes)[258-283]. Increased levels of iron in the body have been linked to the development of hypertension. Iron depletion has also been shown to be protective and also to improve some of the metabolic deficiencies that are characteristic of hypertension. Iron depletion has been demonstrated to be beneficial in lowering the risks of developing cardiovascular disease. Iron depletion may also be beneficial in improving insulin secretion, insulin action and the overall metabolic control in hypertension.

There is no direct evidence that decreasing the intake of dietary iron causes weight loss. To decrease the intake of dietary iron; however, meats and meat products are restricted in the diet. The restriction of meats and meat products is likely to cause weight loss in most people.

The plateau-proof diet for hypertension restricts dietary iron from animal sources but not from plant sources. People who eliminate meats are likely to have greater success than people who restrict meats. Certain fish and other sea food may be substituted for meats. In general though, proteins from plant sources are better than proteins from animal sources for weight control in individuals with hypertension. Proteins from plants sources, such as soy, in addition to affecting a rapid weight loss, may lower the level of glucose in the blood, and increase metabolic control in hypertension.

■

Does increasing the amount of fruits and vegetable in the diet affect weight loss?

Fruits and vegetable are an essential part of a healthy diet. Not all fruits and vegetable; however, are good for weight loss. This is why the plateau-proof diet does not generalize benefits of foods in food groups; rather, each food is assigned a CP and an FP index – numbers that show the individual characteristics of that food.

■

Are there foods that promote weight loss?

Yes there are foods that can promote weight loss. We saw earlier that proteins stimulate thermogenesis, the process where the body gives off energy as heat. It takes energy to generate heat, and the energy is either coming from the diet or from fat stores. In either case the net result is weight loss. This is one of the favorable properties of proteins on which a significant part of the plateau-proof diet is based. The idea however is to make a balanced diet out of foods with low CP and FP indices, rather than to use proteins as a nutritional supplement.

■

Weight loss from cocoa powder?

Recent biomedical studies have shown that cocoa powder can prevent obesity in rats[284]. No parallel studies have been done in humans, but there is a possibility that cocoa powder may contribute to weight loss in humans. Cocoa powder prevents obesity in rats by blocking fat metabolism. Specifically, it suppresses the enzymes (small substances that increase the rate of metabolism and other reactions in the body) that are responsible for making fatty acids. Remember from chapter one that excesses of all macronutrients are stored as triglycerides (fatty acids + glycerol) in fat cells. When the production of fatty acid is blocked by cocoa, there are no triglycerides made; hence no fat stored in the body.

Cocoa powder also increases thermogenesis. We see now that cocoa powder may contribute to weight loss by two distinct mechanisms. If indeed cocoa powder can contribute to weight loss in humans, the idea will be to integrate it into the diet, as part of a balanced diet, while adhering to the principles of the plateau-proof diet.

■

Does increasing calcium intake from dairy affect weight loss?

NO. A recent clinical study showed that increasing calcium in the diet has no effect on weight loss[217]. Additionally, this study showed that short-term weight loss from a hypocaloric high-protein diet is not affected by the source (type) of protein in the diet.

■

Does alcohol have a role in obesity and weight loss?

Recent medical studies have shown that moderate consumption of alcoholic beverages is beneficial for cardiovascular health, amongst other things. Both excessive consumption of alcohol and no consumption of alcohol have been blamed for causing or facilitating diabetes. Although most diet programs discourage the consumption of alcoholic beverages, moderate consumption of alcohol may actually be beneficial to obese subjects. At least one clinical study has shown that moderate consumption of wine does not affect the outcome of weight loss during dieting[285]. Another study involving 334 identical twins showed that the moderate alcohol consuming siblings were leaner than the siblings who abstained from alcohol[286]. Other studies have suggested that consumption of alcohol may contribute to weight loss or may prevent weight gain[287,288].

It should be noted however that excessive consumption of alcohol may cause obesity[289]. Excessive consumption of alcohol may also result in liver disease and cardiovascular disease. In some people, excessive consumption of alcohol may lead to weight loss due to malnutrition[290]. Mindful of the contradicting information on alcohol and weight loss, moderation should be the guiding word for any dieter – moderation in food, moderation in alcohol, and moderation in exercise.

Appendix I

Weight (lbs) / Height (feet) Table

Match your height and your weight. If your weight falls in the white (19 – 24) you are normal, hatch grey (25 – 29) = overweight, and solid grey (above 30) = obese. Below 19 = underweight.

NORMAL						OVERWEIGHT					OBESE			
19	20	21	22	23	24	25	26	27	28	29	30	31	32	
														Height
76	80	84	88	92	96	100	104	108	112	116	120	124	128	4' 5"
79	83	87	91	95	100	104	108	112	116	120	124	129	133	4' 6"
82	86	90	95	99	103	108	112	116	120	125	129	133	138	4' 7"
85	89	94	98	103	107	112	116	120	125	129	134	138	143	4' 8"
88	92	97	102	106	111	116	120	125	129	134	139	143	148	4' 9"
91	96	100	105	110	115	120	124	129	134	139	144	148	153	4' 10"
94	99	104	109	114	119	124	129	134	139	144	149	154	158	4' 11"
97	102	108	113	118	123	128	133	138	143	149	154	159	164	5'
101	106	111	116	122	127	132	138	143	148	153	159	164	169	5' 1"
104	109	115	120	126	131	137	142	148	153	159	164	170	175	5' 2"
107	113	119	124	130	135	141	147	152	158	164	169	175	181	5' 3"
111	117	122	128	134	140	146	151	157	163	169	175	181	186	5' 4"
114	120	126	132	138	144	150	156	162	168	174	180	186	192	5' 5"
118	124	130	136	143	149	155	161	167	173	180	186	192	198	5' 6"
121	128	134	140	147	153	160	166	172	179	185	192	198	204	5' 7"
125	132	138	145	151	158	164	171	178	184	191	197	204	210	5' 8"
129	135	142	149	156	163	169	176	183	190	196	203	210	217	5' 9"
132	139	146	153	160	167	174	181	188	195	202	209	216	223	5' 10"
136	143	151	158	165	172	179	186	194	201	208	215	222	229	5' 11"
140	147	155	162	170	177	184	192	199	206	214	221	229	236	6'
144	152	159	167	174	182	190	197	205	212	220	227	235	243	6' 1"
148	156	164	171	179	187	195	203	210	218	226	234	241	249	6' 2"
152	160	168	176	184	192	200	208	216	224	232	240	248	256	6' 3"
156	164	173	181	189	197	205	214	222	230	238	246	255	263	6' 4"
160	169	177	186	194	202	211	219	228	236	245	253	261	270	6' 5"

164	173	182	190	199	208	216	225	234	242	251	260	268	277	6' 6"
169	178	186	195	204	213	222	231	240	249	257	266	275	284	6' 7"
173	182	191	200	209	218	228	237	246	255	264	273	282	291	6' 8"
177	187	196	205	215	224	233	243	252	261	271	280	289	299	6' 9"
182	191	201	210	220	230	239	249	258	268	277	287	297	306	6' 10"
186	196	206	216	225	235	245	255	265	274	284	294	304	314	6' 11"
191	201	211	221	231	241	251	261	271	281	291	301	311	321	7'
195	206	216	226	236	247	257	267	277	288	298	308	319	329	7' 1"
200	210	221	231	242	252	263	274	284	295	305	316	326	337	7' 2"
205	215	226	237	248	258	269	280	291	301	312	323	334	345	7' 3"
209	220	231	242	253	264	275	286	297	308	319	330	341	353	7' 4"
214	225	237	248	259	270	282	293	304	315	327	338	349	361	7' 5"
219	230	242	253	265	277	288	300	311	323	334	346	357	369	7' 6"

Weight (Kg) / Height (meters) Table

Match your height and your weight. If your weight falls in the white (19 – 24) you are normal, hatch grey (25 – 29) = overweight, and solid grey (above 30) = obese. Below 19 = underweight.

NORMAL						OVERWEIGHT					OBESE			
19	20	21	22	23	24	25	26	27	28	29	30	31	32	
														Height
19	20	21	22	23	24	25	26	27	28	29	30	31	32	1.0
23	24	25	27	28	29	30	31	33	34	35	36	38	39	1.1
27	29	30	32	33	35	36	37	39	40	42	43	45	46	1.2
32	34	35	37	39	41	42	44	46	47	49	51	52	54	1.3
37	39	41	43	45	47	49	51	53	55	57	59	61	63	1.4
43	45	47	50	52	54	56	59	61	63	65	68	70	72	1.5
49	51	54	56	59	61	64	67	69	72	74	77	79	82	1.6
55	58	61	64	66	69	72	75	78	81	84	87	90	92	1.7
62	65	68	71	75	78	81	84	87	91	94	97	100	104	1.8
69	72	76	79	83	87	90	94	97	101	105	108	112	116	1.9
76	80	84	88	92	96	100	104	108	112	116	120	124	128	2.0
84	88	93	97	101	106	110	115	119	123	128	132	137	141	2.1
92	97	102	106	111	116	121	126	131	136	140	145	150	155	2.2
101	106	111	116	122	127	132	138	143	148	153	159	164	169	2.3
109	115	121	127	132	138	144	150	156	161	167	173	179	184	2.4
119	125	131	138	144	150	156	163	169	175	181	188	194	200	2.5
128	135	142	149	155	162	169	176	183	189	196	203	210	216	2.6
139	146	153	160	168	175	182	190	197	204	211	219	226	233	2.7
149	157	165	172	180	188	196	204	212	220	227	235	243	251	2.8
160	168	177	185	193	202	210	219	227	235	244	252	261	269	2.9
171	180	189	198	207	216	225	234	243	252	261	270	279	288	3.0

Appendix II

Sample ~ 400g (~14.1 oz) per day CP menu

Breakfast – Ham omelet
2 eggs
Turkey ham – 1oz
Yogurt (nonfat) – 2 oz
Coffee or tea (unsweetened)

Lunch – Chicken roll and salad
Baked sole – 3 oz
Tossed greens – 3 cups
Ranch dressing – 3 tablespoons
Walnuts – 1 oz

Dinner – Steak and shrimp
Sirloin steak – 4 oz
Shrimp – 1 oz
Carrots – 0.5 oz
Green beans – 0.5 oz

■

Sample ~ 400g (~14.1 oz) per day FP menu

Breakfast – Cereal and fruit
All-bran cereal in nonfat milk – 3 oz
Strawberries – 1 oz

Lunch – Ham sandwich
Turkey ham (lean) – 2 oz
2 slices of bread
Baked potato chips – 1 oz

Dinner – Grilled salmon and baked potato
Grilled salmon – 4 oz
1 small baked potato
Kiwi fruit – 2 oz

Bibliography

1. Izmozherova, N.V. et al. [Arterial hypertension, disorders of carbohydrate and lipid metabolism in obese perimenopausal females]. *Ter Arkh* **77**, 67-9 (2005).

2. Fuh, M.M., Shieh, S.M., Wu, D.A., Chen, Y.D. & Reaven, G.M. Abnormalities of carbohydrate and lipid metabolism in patients with hypertension. *Arch Intern Med* **147**, 1035-8 (1987).

3. Singer, P., Baumann, R., Voigt, S. & Godicke, W. [Clinical aspects of typical changes in carbohydrate and lipid metabolism in essential hypertension]. *Z Gesamte Inn Med* **37**, 325-30 (1982).

4. Baumann, R. [Disorders of carbohydrate and lipid metabolism in the early stages of essential hypertension as the pathogenetic factors of arteriosclerosis risk]. *Vestn Akad Med Nauk SSSR*, 76-87 (1977).

5. Baumann, R. [Carbohydrate and lipid metabolism disorders in early stages of essential hypertension as pathogenetic risk factors of arteriosclerosis]. *Z Gesamte Inn Med* **28**, 193-201 concl (1973).

6. Shizuka, K. & Yambe, T. [Relationship between depression and lipid metabolism in the elderly with hypertension]. *Nippon Ronen Igakkai Zasshi* **38**, 785-90 (2001).

7.   Cia Gomez, P., Martinez-Berganza, A., Cia Blasco, P., Mozota Duarte, J. & Marin Ballve, A. [Arterial hypertension and lipid metabolism]. *An Med Interna* **16**, 315-20 (1999).

8.   Zicha, J., Kunes, J. & Devynck, M.A. Abnormalities of membrane function and lipid metabolism in hypertension: a review. *Am J Hypertens* **12**, 315-31 (1999).

9.   Agata, J. et al. Association of insulin resistance and hyperinsulinemia with disturbed lipid metabolism in patients with essential hypertension. *Hypertens Res* **21**, 57-62 (1998).

10.   Lopes, H.F. et al. Lipid metabolism alterations in normotensive subjects with positive family history of hypertension. *Hypertension* **30**, 629-31 (1997).

11.   Clemenzia, G. et al. Hypertension and CHD: evidence of glucose and lipid metabolism involvement. *Riv Eur Sci Med Farmacol* **18**, 105-11 (1996).

12.   Pannier, B.M. et al. Abnormalities of lipid metabolism and arterial rigidity in young subjects with borderline hypertension. *Clin Invest Med* **17**, 42-51 (1994).

13.   Kistler, T. & Weisser, B. [Correlation between disorders of lipid metabolism and hypertension in 10,892 participants in the Heureka Study]. *Schweiz Rundsch Med Prax* **82**, 1222-33 (1993).

14.   Titkov Iu, S. [Disordered lipid metabolism in patients with arterial hypertension]. *Vrach Delo*, 53-5 (1991).

15. Mazo, R.Z. & Korol, S.M. [The characteristics of lipid metabolism in children with primary arterial hypertension]. *Pediatriia*, 8-11 (1991).

16. Krawczuk-Rybakowa, M., Maslowiecka, J., Urban, M. & Siwinski, J. [Evaluation of selected parameters of lipid metabolism in children with arterial hypertension]. *Kardiol Pol* **31**, 180-5 (1988).

17. Samsonov, M.A., Krylov, V.I. & Medvedeva, I.A. [Effect of fat loading on indicators of lipid metabolism in hypertension]. *Sov Med*, 5-8 (1986).

18. Mikheeva, V.A. [Various indices of lipid metabolism in children and adolescents in the risk group for inheritance of hypertension]. *Pediatriia*, 67-8 (1983).

19. Aleksenko, A.S., Bel'chenko, D.I., Volkov, V.S., Andreianova, G.N. & Anikin, V.V. [Arterial hypertension and atherogenic disorders of lipid metabolism]. *Klin Med (Mosk)* **56**, 111-8 (1978).

20. Barbulescu, A. & Suteanu, S. [Disorders of lipid metabolism in essential arterial hypertension in young people]. *Med Interna (Bucur)* **25**, 711-24 (1973).

21. Ubaidullaev, A.M. & Bavina, M.B. [Changes in lipid metabolism in various forms of arterial hypertension]. *Kardiologiia* **13**, 62-6 (1973).

22. Studenikin, M. & Abdullaev, A.R. [Some indices of lipid metabolism in children and adolescents with hypertension]. *Vopr Okhr Materin Det* **14**, 44-8 (1969).

23.   Kreze, A. [Interrelationship between obesity and hypertension. II. Indices of lipid metabolism]. *Bratisl Lek Listy* **50**, 499-506 (1968).

24.   Priss, I.S. [Some features of lipid metabolism changes in uncomplicated hypertension.]. *Sov Med* **22**, 9-19 (1958).

25.   Otani, H. [Pathophysiological Study on Cerebral Carbohydrate Metabolism in Essential Hypertension and Cerebral Arteriosclerosis. 1. Study on Cerebral Carbohydrate Metabolism During Rest.]. *Jpn Circ J* **27**, 534-46 (1963).

26.   Baumann, R. & Graff, C. [Association of early-stage essential hypertension with latent asymptomatic diabetic carbohydrate metabolism disorders. I]. *Dtsch Gesundheitsw* **23**, 1585-93 (1968).

27.   Simonian, A.T. & Bostandzhian, O. [Effect of hypothiazide on carbohydrate metabolism in patients with diabetes mellitus and hypertension]. *Ter Arkh* **41**, 77-81 (1969).

28.   Luthy, R. [Study of serum lipids in normal persons and patients with essential hypertension with reference to carbohydrate metabolism]. *Praxis* **58**, 1365-72 contd (1969).

29.   Luthy, R. [Studies of serum lipids in healthy subjects and patients with essential hypertension with reference to carbohydrate metabolism. II]. *Praxis* **58**, 1413-23 (1969).

30.   Singer, P., Zimmermann, H.B. & Gawellek, F. [Studies on the carbohydrate metabolism in renovascular and essential hypertension with consideration of thiazide therapy]. *Dtsch Z Verdau Stoffwechselkr* **30**, 185-200 (1970).

31. Singer, P., Honigmann, G. & Dubrau, B. [Serum lipids in renal artery stenosis and essential hypertension with reference to carbohydrate metabolism]. *Z Gesamte Inn Med* **26**, 522-7 passim (1971).

32. Pretolani, E. & Zoli, I. [Hypertension and disorder of carbohydrate metabolism]. *Nouv Presse Med* **1**, 2692 (1972).

33. Zoli, I. et al. [Hypertension and carbohydrate metabolism disorders]. *Cardiol Prat* **24**, 171-6 (1973).

34. Nadal de los Santos Reyes, M., Montis Suau, R. & Sastre Alzamora, P. [Sella turcica, arterial hypertension and carbohydrate metabolism in obesity: statistical study of 100 cases]. *Rev Clin Esp* **160**, 327-30 (1981).

35. Ruiatkina, L.A., Dikker, V.E. & Galenok, V.A. [Early diagnosis of carbohydrate metabolism disorders in patients with essential hypertension]. *Klin Med (Mosk)* **65**, 113-8 (1987).

36. Reaven, G.M. & Hoffman, B.B. Abnormalities of carbohydrate metabolism may play a role in the etiology and clinical course of hypertension. *Trends Pharmacol Sci* **9**, 78-9 (1988).

37. Sowers, J.R., Standley, P.R., Ram, J.L., Zemel, M.B. & Resnick, L.M. Insulin resistance, carbohydrate metabolism, and hypertension. *Am J Hypertens* **4**, 466S-472S (1991).

38. Gambardella, S. et al. Carbohydrate metabolism in hypertension: influence of treatment. *J Cardiovasc Pharmacol* **22 Suppl 6**, S87-97 (1993).

39. Sechi, L.A., Catena, C., Zingaro, L., De Carli, S. & Bartoli, E. Hypertension and abnormalities of carbohydrate metabolism possible role of the sympathetic nervous system. *Am J Hypertens* **10**, 678-82 (1997).

40. Kobalava Zh, D. et al. [Clinicogenetic aspects of carbohydrate metabolism disorders and efficacy of their correction with moxonidine and metformine in patients with arterial hypertension]. *Ter Arkh* **77**, 46-51 (2005).

41. Kobalava, Z.D. et al. [Clinical Genetic Determinants of Carbohydrate Metabolism Disturbances in Patients With Hypertension and Excessive Weight.]. *Kardiologiia* **45**, 37-43 (2005).

42. Parillo, M., Coulston, A., Hollenbeck, C. & Reaven, G. Effect of a low fat diet on carbohydrate metabolism in patients with hypertension. *Hypertension* **11**, 244-8 (1988).

43. Alagille, D. [Diabetes: review of glucose metabolism and the physiopathology of diabetes.]. *Vie Med* **35**, 683-8 (1954).

44. Anderson, J.W. Recent advances in carbohydrate nutrition and metabolism in diabetes mellitus. *J Am Coll Nutr* **8 Suppl**, 61S-67S (1989).

45. Basu, A., Shah, P., Nielsen, M., Basu, R. & Rizza, R.A. Effects of type 2 diabetes on the regulation of hepatic glucose metabolism. *J Investig Med* **52**, 366-74 (2004).

46. Betteridge, D.J. Diabetes, lipoprotein metabolism and atherosclerosis. *Br Med Bull* **45**, 285-311 (1989).

47.   Bierman, E.L. [Diabetes in the pathogenesis of atherosclerosis--
        a background disturbance in lipid metabolism]. *Duodecim* **105**,
        1469-74 (1989).

48.   Biesenbach, G. [Disorders of lipid metabolism in diabetes
        mellitus]. *Wien Med Wochenschr Suppl* **105**, 9-17 (1989).

49.   Blaak, E.E. Fatty acid metabolism in obesity and type 2
        diabetes mellitus. *Proc Nutr Soc* **62**, 753-60 (2003).

50.   Blaak, E.E. Basic disturbances in skeletal muscle fatty acid
        metabolism in obesity and type 2 diabetes mellitus. *Proc Nutr
        Soc* **63**, 323-30 (2004).

51.   Boden, G. Effects of free fatty acids (FFA) on glucose
        metabolism: significance for insulin resistance and type 2
        diabetes. *Exp Clin Endocrinol Diabetes* **111**, 121-4 (2003).

52.   Bonadonna, R.C. & De Fronzo, R.A. Glucose metabolism in
        obesity and type 2 diabetes. *Diabete Metab* **17**, 112-35 (1991).

53.   Bonadonna, R.C. Alterations of glucose metabolism in type 2
        diabetes mellitus. An overview. *Rev Endocr Metab Disord* **5**,
        89-97 (2004).

54.   Bonanome, A. et al. Carbohydrate and lipid metabolism in
        patients with non-insulin-dependent diabetes mellitus: effects of
        a low-fat, high-carbohydrate diet vs a diet high in
        monounsaturated fatty acids. *Am J Clin Nutr* **54**, 586-90 (1991).

55.   Bremer, J. [The metabolism of fatty acids in diabetes]. *Tidsskr
        Nor Laegeforen* **91**, 1296-8 (1971).

56.   Cardonnet, L.J. [Lipid metabolism in diabetes]. *Rev Argent Endocrinol Metab* **14**, 57-64 (1968).

57.   Carmena, R. & Grande, F. [Changes of lipid metabolism in diabetes mellitus]. *Rev Clin Esp* **108**, 85-99 (1968).

58.   Dinneen, S., Gerich, J. & Rizza, R. Carbohydrate metabolism in non-insulin-dependent diabetes mellitus. *N Engl J Med* **327**, 707-13 (1992).

59.   Georgopoulos, A. Postprandial triglyceride metabolism in diabetes mellitus. *Clin Cardiol* **22**, II28-33 (1999).

60.   Ginsberg, H.N. Very low density lipoprotein metabolism in diabetes mellitus. *Diabetes Metab Rev* **3**, 571-89 (1987).

61.   Girard, J. [Biochemical bases of abnormalities of glucose metabolism in non-insulin-dependent diabetes]. *Journ Annu Diabetol Hotel Dieu*, 81-96 (1993).

62.   Gordon, E.S. Lipid Metabolism, Diabetes Mellitus, and Obesity. *Adv Intern Med* **12**, 66-102 (1964).

63.   Goto, Y. [Metabolism of various carbohydrates in diabetes mellitus]. *Nippon Rinsho* **25**, 261-7 (1967).

64.   Hallfrisch, J. Dietary sugars and carbohydrate metabolism in type II diabetes. *J Am Coll Nutr* **6**, 385-96 (1987).

65.   Hopp, H., Leis, R. & Albus, C. [Changes in carbohydrate and lipid metabolism and modification of diabetes mellitus by

hormonal contraceptives]. *Z Arztl Fortbild (Jena)* **84**, 31-4 (1990).

66. Hother-Nielsen, O. & Beck-Nielsen, H. Basal glucose metabolism in type 2 diabetes. A critical review. *Diabete Metab* **17**, 136-45 (1991).

67. Howard, B.V. Lipoprotein metabolism in diabetes mellitus. *J Lipid Res* **28**, 613-28 (1987).

68. Howard, B.V. Lipoprotein metabolism in diabetes. *Curr Opin Lipidol* **5**, 216-20 (1994).

69. Iizuka, Y. & Murase, T. [Abnormalities in lipid metabolism associated with diabetes mellitus]. *Nippon Rinsho* **55 Suppl**, 603-8 (1997).

70. Joven, J., Vilella, E. & Masana, L. [Metabolism of lipoproteins in diabetes mellitus]. *Med Clin (Barc)* **93**, 752-5 (1989).

71. Kamysheva, E.P., Bushueva, G.V., Gorovaia, V.I., Maslennikova, G.V. & Mashkova, T.N. [Carbohydrate metabolism disorders in diabetes mellitus patients]. *Ter Arkh* **43**, 60-3 (1971).

72. Kawahara, R. [Diabetes mellitus and lipid metabolism]. *Rinsho Byori* **35**, 847-52 (1987).

73. Keenan, B.S. et al. The effect of diet upon carbohydrate metabolism, insulin resistance, and blood pressure in congenital total lipoatrophic diabetes. *Metabolism* **29**, 1214-24 (1980).

74.   Kissebah, A.H. Low density lipoprotein metabolism in non-insulin-dependent diabetes mellitus. *Diabetes Metab Rev* **3**, 619-51 (1987).

75.   Klip, A. et al. Effect of diabetes on glucoregulation. From glucose transporters to glucose metabolism in vivo. *Diabetes Care* **15**, 1747-66 (1992).

76.   Kuwajima, M., Shima, K. & Matsuyama, T. [Abnormal carbohydrate metabolism in diabetes mellitus]. *Nippon Rinsho* **55 Suppl**, 593-601 (1997).

77.   Kuwajima, M. [Disorder of carbohydrate metabolism in diabetes]. *Nippon Rinsho* **60 Suppl 8**, 139-44 (2002).

78.   Leites, S.M. [Fat-Lipid Metabolism in Diabetes Mellitus.]. *Probl Endokrinol Gormonoter* **18**, 3-12 (1963).

79.   Leites, S.M. [Pathogenesis of lipid metabolism disorders in diabetes mellitus]. *Ter Arkh* **44**, 16-22 (1972).

80.   Lewis, G.F. Postprandial lipoprotein metabolism in diabetes mellitus and obesity. *J Atheroscler Thromb* **2 Suppl 1**, S34-5 (1995).

81.   Lopes-Virella, M.F. [Metabolism of lipoproteins in diabetes mellitus]. *Journ Annu Diabetol Hotel Dieu*, 55-66 (1987).

82.   Martin, I.K. & Wahren, J. Glucose metabolism during physical exercise in patients with noninsulin-dependent (type II) diabetes. *Adv Exp Med Biol* **334**, 221-33 (1993).

83. McCall, A.L. Cerebral glucose metabolism in diabetes mellitus. *Eur J Pharmacol* **490**, 147-58 (2004).

84. McGarry, J.D. Disordered metabolism in diabetes: have we underemphasized the fat component? *J Cell Biochem* **55 Suppl**, 29-38 (1994).

85. Mero, N., Syvanne, M. & Taskinen, M.R. Postprandial lipid metabolism in diabetes. *Atherosclerosis* **141 Suppl 1**, S53-5 (1998).

86. Meyer, C. & Schwaiger, M. Myocardial blood flow and glucose metabolism in diabetes mellitus. *Am J Cardiol* **80**, 94A-101A (1997).

87. Mincu, I. & Georgescu, S. [Metabolism of Lipids in Diabetes.]. *Med Interna (Bucur)* **16**, 1209-26 (1964).

88. Mudrikova, T., Tkac, I. & Takac, M. [Changes in lipoprotein metabolism in patients with diabetes mellitus and the effect on lipid profile in diabetics]. *Vnitr Lek* **40**, 250-4 (1994).

89. Murakami, M., Sekimoto, H., Yasuda, Y., Masuda, S. & Genda, A. [Lipid metabolism in diabetes mellitus]. *Saishin Igaku* **20**, 1639-48 (1965).

90. Nikkila, E.A. Triglyceride metabolism in diabetes mellitus. *Prog Biochem Pharmacol* **8**, 271-99 (1973).

91. Nikkila, E.A. Very low density lipoprotein triglyceride metabolism in diabetes. *Monogr Atheroscler* **13**, 44-52 (1985).

92. Poisson, J.P. Essential fatty acid metabolism in diabetes. *Nutrition* **5**, 263-6 (1989).

93. Murphy, N.J. et al. Hypertension in Alaska Natives: association with overweight, glucose intolerance, diet and mechanized activity. *Ethn Health* **2**, 267-75 (1997).

94. Dunaeva, T.M., Milovidova, S.S. & Bogoliubov, V.M. [Reducing-diet therapy of patients with arterial hypertension associated with alimentary obesity]. *Sov Med*, 106-9 (1976).

95. Young, J.B. & Landsberg, L. Diet-induced changes in sympathetic nervous system activity: possible implications for obesity and hypertension. *J Chronic Dis* **35**, 879-86 (1982).

96. Douglass, J.M. et al. Effects of a raw food diet on hypertension and obesity. *South Med J* **78**, 841-4 (1985).

97. Singh, R.B. et al. Effect of low energy diet and weight loss on major risk factors, central obesity and associated disturbances in patients with essential hypertension. *J Hum Hypertens* **9**, 355-62 (1995).

98. Pecelj-Gec, M., Jorga, J., Rsumovic, S., Neradovic-Mladenovski, L. & Zbutega-Milosevic, G. Effects of reducing diet and increased leisure time physical activity on hypertension associated with obesity. *Acta Med Iugosl* **44**, 367-76 (1990).

99. Beegom, R., Niaz, M.A. & Singh, R.B. Diet, central obesity and prevalence of hypertension in the urban population of south India. *Int J Cardiol* **51**, 183-91 (1995).

100. Heyden, S. The workinghman's diet. II. Effect of weight reduction in obese patients with hypertension, diabetes, hyperuricemia and hyperlipidemia. *Nutr Metab* **22**, 141-59 (1978).

101. Singh, R.B., Rastogi, S.S., Mehta, P.J., Mody, R. & Garg, V. Effect of diet and weight reduction in hypertension. *Nutrition* **6**, 297-302 (1990).

102. Boden, G., Sargrad, K., Homko, C., Mozzoli, M. & Stein, T.P. Effect of a low-carbohydrate diet on appetite, blood glucose levels, and insulin resistance in obese patients with type 2 diabetes. *Ann Intern Med* **142**, 403-11 (2005).

103. Groop, L.C., Widen, E. & Ferrannini, E. Insulin resistance and insulin deficiency in the pathogenesis of type 2 (non-insulin-dependent) diabetes mellitus: errors of metabolism or of methods? *Diabetologia* **36**, 1326-31 (1993).

104. Koffler, M. & Kisch, E.S. Starvation diet and very-low-calorie diets may induce insulin resistance and overt diabetes mellitus. *J Diabetes Complications* **10**, 109-12 (1996).

105. Pedersen, O., Hermansen, K., Palmvig, B., Pedersen, S.E. & Sondergaard, K. [Diabetes and diet--changes in insulin resistance induced by food and need of individualized dietary guidelines]. *Ugeskr Laeger* **154**, 2573-4 (1992).

106. Efremov, A.V. et al. [The specificity of lipid metabolism in hereditary arterial hypertension induced by stress]. *Klin Lab Diagn*, 14-6 (2000).

107. Man, Z.W., Hirashima, T., Mori, S. & Kawano, K. Decrease in triglyceride accumulation in tissues by restricted diet and improvement of diabetes in Otsuka Long-Evans Tokushima fatty rats, a non-insulin-dependent diabetes model. *Metabolism* **49**, 108-14 (2000).

108. De Man, F.H., Cabezas, M.C., Van Barlingen, H.H., Erkelens, D.W. & de Bruin, T.W. Triglyceride-rich lipoproteins in non-insulin-dependent diabetes mellitus: post-prandial metabolism and relation to premature atherosclerosis. *Eur J Clin Invest* **26**, 89-108 (1996).

109. Bogatyreva Sh, I., Dzeranova, N. & Zaripova, Z. [Free fatty acid and triglyceride content of the blood in newly-detected diabetes mellitus with prolonged preservation of normoglycemia as a result of diet therapy in combination with sulfanilamide antidiabetic preparations]. *Probl Endokrinol (Mosk)* **19**, 3-7 (1973).

110. Suzuki, S. [Abnormalities of amino acid metabolism in diabetes mellitus]. *Nippon Rinsho* **55 Suppl**, 625-9 (1997).

111. Newsholme, P., Brennan, L., Rubi, B. & Maechler, P. New insights into amino acid metabolism, beta-cell function and diabetes. *Clin Sci (Lond)* **108**, 185-94 (2005).

112. Darmaun, D. [Insulin, diabetes, and amino acid metabolism]. *Journ Annu Diabetol Hotel Dieu*, 105-15 (2002).

113. Abu-Lebdeh, H.S. & Nair, K.S. Protein metabolism in diabetes mellitus. *Baillieres Clin Endocrinol Metab* **10**, 589-601 (1996).

114. Bodnar, P.N. [Protein metabolism indices in diabetes mellitus patients (review of the literature)]. *Vrach Delo* **11**, 96-9 (1972).

115. Brinkworth, G.D., Noakes, M., Parker, B., Foster, P. & Clifton, P.M. Long-term effects of advice to consume a high-protein, low-fat diet, rather than a conventional weight-loss diet, in obese adults with type 2 diabetes: one-year follow-up of a randomised trial. *Diabetologia* **47**, 1677-86 (2004).

116. De Feo, P. Fed state protein metabolism in diabetes mellitus. *J Nutr* **128**, 328S-332S (1998).

117. Gannon, M.C. & Nuttall, F.Q. Effect of a high-protein, low-carbohydrate diet on blood glucose control in people with type 2 diabetes. *Diabetes* **53**, 2375-82 (2004).

118. Hilton, A.D. & Hursh, T.A. Type 2 diabetes in an aviator, protein diet vs. traditional diet: case report. *Aviat Space Environ Med* **72**, 219-20 (2001).

119. Parker, B., Noakes, M., Luscombe, N. & Clifton, P. Effect of a high-protein, high-monounsaturated fat weight loss diet on glycemic control and lipid levels in type 2 diabetes. *Diabetes Care* **25**, 425-30 (2002).

120. Seino, Y., Seino, S., Ikeda, M., Matsukura, S. & Imura, H. Beneficial effects of high protein diet in treatment of mild diabetes. *Hum Nutr Appl Nutr* **37 A**, 226-30 (1983).

121. Tessari, P. Amino acid and protein metabolism in diabetes mellitus. *Ital J Gastroenterol* **25**, 151-5 (1993).

122. Tessari, P., Barazzoni, R., Zanetti, M., Kiwanuka, E. & Tiengo, A. Protein metabolism in Type 1 and Type 2 diabetes mellitus in the fasted and fed states. *Diabetes Nutr Metab* **12**, 428-34 (1999).

123. Beilin, L.J. & Burke, V. Vegetarian diet components, protein and blood pressure: which nutrients are important? *Clin Exp Pharmacol Physiol* **22**, 195-8 (1995).

124. Nobels, F., van Gaal, L. & de Leeuw, I. Weight reduction with a high protein, low carbohydrate, calorie-restricted diet: effects on blood pressure, glucose and insulin levels. *Neth J Med* **35**, 295-302 (1989).

125. Nuttall, F.Q., Gannon, M.C., Saeed, A., Jordan, K. & Hoover, H. The metabolic response of subjects with type 2 diabetes to a high-protein, weight-maintenance diet. *J Clin Endocrinol Metab* **88**, 3577-83 (2003).

126. Nuttall, F.Q. & Gannon, M.C. Metabolic response of people with type 2 diabetes to a high protein diet. *Nutr Metab (Lond)* **1**, 6 (2004).

127. Wing, R.R., Blair, E., Marcus, M., Epstein, L.H. & Harvey, J. Year-long weight loss treatment for obese patients with type II diabetes: does including an intermittent very-low-calorie diet improve outcome? *Am J Med* **97**, 354-62 (1994).

128. Heilbronn, L.K., Noakes, M. & Clifton, P.M. Effect of energy restriction, weight loss, and diet composition on plasma lipids and glucose in patients with type 2 diabetes. *Diabetes Care* **22**, 889-95 (1999).

129. Meckling, K.A., O'Sullivan, C. & Saari, D. Comparison of a low-fat diet to a low-carbohydrate diet on weight loss, body composition, and risk factors for diabetes and cardiovascular disease in free-living, overweight men and women. *J Clin Endocrinol Metab* **89**, 2717-23 (2004).

130. Paisey, R.B. et al. Five year results of a prospective very low calorie diet or conventional weight loss programme in type 2 diabetes. *J Hum Nutr Diet* **15**, 121-7 (2002).

131. Tong, P.C. et al. The effect of orlistat-induced weight loss, without concomitant hypocaloric diet, on cardiovascular risk factors and insulin sensitivity in young obese Chinese subjects with or without type 2 diabetes. *Arch Intern Med* **162**, 2428-35 (2002).

132. Williams, K.V. & Kelley, D.E. Metabolic consequences of weight loss on glucose metabolism and insulin action in type 2 diabetes. *Diabetes Obes Metab* **2**, 121-9 (2000).

133. Ryttig, K.R., Flaten, H. & Rossner, S. Long-term effects of a very low calorie diet (Nutrilett) in obesity treatment. A prospective, randomized, comparison between VLCD and a hypocaloric diet+behavior modification and their combination. *Int J Obes Relat Metab Disord* **21**, 574-9 (1997).

134. Blanch Miro, S., Recasens Gracia, M.A., Sola Alberich, R. & Salas-Salvado, J. [Effect of a highly hypocaloric diet on the control of morbid obesity in the short and the long term]. *Med Clin (Barc)* **100**, 450-3 (1993).

135. Coleman, M.D. & Nickols-Richardson, S.M. Urinary ketones reflect serum ketone concentration but do not relate to weight

loss in overweight premenopausal women following a low-carbohydrate/high-protein diet. *J Am Diet Assoc* **105**, 608-11 (2005).

136.   Foster, G.D. et al. A randomized trial of a low-carbohydrate diet for obesity. *N Engl J Med* **348**, 2082-90 (2003).

137.   Meckling, K.A., Gauthier, M., Grubb, R. & Sanford, J. Effects of a hypocaloric, low-carbohydrate diet on weight loss, blood lipids, blood pressure, glucose tolerance, and body composition in free-living overweight women. *Can J Physiol Pharmacol* **80**, 1095-105 (2002).

138.   Samaha, F.F. et al. A low-carbohydrate as compared with a low-fat diet in severe obesity. *N Engl J Med* **348**, 2074-81 (2003).

139.   Seshadri, P. et al. A randomized study comparing the effects of a low-carbohydrate diet and a conventional diet on lipoprotein subfractions and C-reactive protein levels in patients with severe obesity. *Am J Med* **117**, 398-405 (2004).

140.   Stern, L. et al. The effects of low-carbohydrate versus conventional weight loss diets in severely obese adults: one-year follow-up of a randomized trial. *Ann Intern Med* **140**, 778-85 (2004).

141.   Dessein, P.H., Shipton, E.A., Stanwix, A.E., Joffe, B.I. & Ramokgadi, J. Beneficial effects of weight loss associated with moderate calorie/carbohydrate restriction, and increased proportional intake of protein and unsaturated fat on serum urate and lipoprotein levels in gout: a pilot study. *Ann Rheum Dis* **59**, 539-43 (2000).

142.   Layman, D.K. et al. A reduced ratio of dietary carbohydrate to protein improves body composition and blood lipid profiles during weight loss in adult women. *J Nutr* **133**, 411-7 (2003).

143.   Lean, M.E., Han, T.S., Prvan, T., Richmond, P.R. & Avenell, A. Weight loss with high and low carbohydrate 1200 kcal diets in free living women. *Eur J Clin Nutr* **51**, 243-8 (1997).

144.   Miyashita, Y. et al. Beneficial effect of low carbohydrate in low calorie diets on visceral fat reduction in type 2 diabetic patients with obesity. *Diabetes Res Clin Pract* **65**, 235-41 (2004).

145.   Hauner, H. [Low-carbohydrate or low-fat diet for weight loss--which is better?]. *MMW Fortschr Med* **146**, 33-5, 37 (2004).

146.   Johnston, C.S., Tjonn, S.L. & Swan, P.D. High-protein, low-fat diets are effective for weight loss and favorably alter biomarkers in healthy adults. *J Nutr* **134**, 586-91 (2004).

147.   Bahadori, B. et al. Low-fat, high-carbohydrate (low-glycaemic index) diet induces weight loss and preserves lean body mass in obese healthy subjects: results of a 24-week study. *Diabetes Obes Metab* **7**, 290-3 (2005).

148.   Moyad, M.A. Fad diets and obesity--Part IV: Low-carbohydrate vs. low-fat diets. *Urol Nurs* **25**, 67-70 (2005).

149.   Noakes, M., Keogh, J.B., Foster, P.R. & Clifton, P.M. Effect of an energy-restricted, high-protein, low-fat diet relative to a conventional high-carbohydrate, low-fat diet on weight loss, body composition, nutritional status, and markers of cardiovascular health in obese women. *Am J Clin Nutr* **81**, 1298-306 (2005).

150. Sharman, M.J. & Volek, J.S. Weight loss leads to reductions in inflammatory biomarkers after a very-low-carbohydrate diet and a low-fat diet in overweight men. *Clin Sci (Lond)* **107**, 365-9 (2004).

151. Volek, J. et al. Comparison of energy-restricted very low-carbohydrate and low-fat diets on weight loss and body composition in overweight men and women. *Nutr Metab (Lond)* **1**, 13 (2004).

152. Willi, S.M., Oexmann, M.J., Wright, N.M., Collop, N.A. & Key, L.L., Jr. The effects of a high-protein, low-fat, ketogenic diet on adolescents with morbid obesity: body composition, blood chemistries, and sleep abnormalities. *Pediatrics* **101**, 61-7 (1998).

153. Yancy, W.S., Jr., Olsen, M.K., Guyton, J.R., Bakst, R.P. & Westman, E.C. A low-carbohydrate, ketogenic diet versus a low-fat diet to treat obesity and hyperlipidemia: a randomized, controlled trial. *Ann Intern Med* **140**, 769-77 (2004).

154. Benoit, F.L., Martin, R.L. & Watten, R.H. Changes in body composition during weight reduction in obesity. Balance studies comparing effects of fasting and a ketogenic diet. *Ann Intern Med* **63**, 604-12 (1965).

155. Vazquez, J.A. & Adibi, S.A. Protein sparing during treatment of obesity: ketogenic versus nonketogenic very low calorie diet. *Metabolism* **41**, 406-14 (1992).

156. Van Itallie, T.B. Dietary fiber and obesity. *Am J Clin Nutr* **31**, S43-52 (1978).

157.   Ullrich, I.H. & Albrink, M.J. The effect of dietary fiber and other factors on insulin response: role in obesity. *J Environ Pathol Toxicol Oncol* **5**, 137-55 (1985).

158.   Trallero Casanas, R. [Fiber in the treatment of obesity and its comorbidities]. *Nutr Hosp* **17 Suppl 1**, 17-22 (2002).

159.   Southgate, D.A. Has dietary fibre a role in the prevention and treatment of obesity. *Bibl Nutr Dieta*, 70-6 (1978).

160.   Smith, U. Dietary fibre, diabetes and obesity. *Int J Obes* **11 Suppl 1**, 27-31 (1987).

161.   Silman, A.J. Cereal fibre, total energy intake, and obesity. *Lancet* **2**, 905 (1979).

162.   Leeds, A.R. Treatment of obesity with dietary fibre: present position and potential developments. *Scand J Gastroenterol Suppl* **129**, 156-8 (1987).

163.   Kimm, S.Y. The role of dietary fiber in the development and treatment of childhood obesity. *Pediatrics* **96**, 1010-4 (1995).

164.   Kaul, L. & Nidiry, J. High-fiber diet in the treatment of obesity and hypercholesterolemia. *J Natl Med Assoc* **85**, 231-2 (1993).

165.   Gropper, S.S. & Acosta, P.B. The therapeutic effect of fiber in treating obesity. *J Am Coll Nutr* **6**, 533-5 (1987).

166.   Baron, J.A., Schori, A., Crow, B., Carter, R. & Mann, J.I. A randomized controlled trial of low carbohydrate and low

fat/high fiber diets for weight loss. *Am J Public Health* **76**, 1293-6 (1986).

167. Andersson, B., Terning, K. & Bjorntorp, P. Dietary treatment of obesity localized in different regions. The effect of dietary fibre on relapse. *Int J Obes* **11 Suppl 1**, 79-85 (1987).

168. Anderson, J.W. & Bryant, C.A. Dietary fiber: diabetes and obesity. *Am J Gastroenterol* **81**, 898-906 (1986).

169. Albrink, M.J. Dietary fiber, plasma insulin, and obesity. *Am J Clin Nutr* **31**, S277-S279 (1978).

170. Kritchevsky, D. & Story, J.A. Dietary fiber and cancer. *Curr Concepts Nutr* **6**, 41-54 (1977).

171. Burkitt, D.P. Colonic-rectal cancer: fiber and other dietary factors. *Am J Clin Nutr* **31**, S58-S64 (1978).

172. Esser, W., Weithofer, G. & Bloch, R. [The significance of dietary fat and fiber for the aetiology of colon cancer (author's transl)]. *Z Gastroenterol* **18**, 30-7 (1980).

173. Talbot, J.M. Role of dietary fiber in diverticular disease and colon cancer. *Fed Proc* **40**, 2337-42 (1981).

174. Kritchevsky, D. Dietary fiber and cancer. *Nutr Cancer* **6**, 213-9 (1984).

175. Bright-See, E. et al. Dietary fiber and cancer: a supplement for intervention studies. *Nutr Cancer* **7**, 211-20 (1985).

176. Greenwald, P. & Lanza, E. Role of dietary fiber in the prevention of cancer. *Important Adv Oncol*, 37-54 (1986).

177. Klurfeld, D.M. & Kritchevsky, D. Dietary fiber and human cancer: critique of the literature. *Adv Exp Med Biol* **206**, 119-35 (1986).

178. Jacobs, L.R. Relationship between dietary fiber and cancer: metabolic, physiologic, and cellular mechanisms. *Proc Soc Exp Biol Med* **183**, 299-310 (1986).

179. Ho, E.E., Atwood, J.R. & Meyskens, F.L., Jr. Methodological development of dietary fiber intervention to lower colon cancer risk. *Prog Clin Biol Res* **248**, 263-81 (1987).

180. Burkitt, D.P. Dietary fiber and cancer. *J Nutr* **118**, 531-3 (1988).

181. Rose, D.P. Dietary fiber and breast cancer. *Nutr Cancer* **13**, 1-8 (1990).

182. Cheah, P.Y. & Bernstein, H. Colon cancer and dietary fiber: cellulose inhibits the DNA-damaging ability of bile acids. *Nutr Cancer* **13**, 51-7 (1990).

183. Ross, J.K., Pusateri, D.J. & Shultz, T.D. Dietary and hormonal evaluation of men at different risks for prostate cancer: fiber intake, excretion, and composition, with in vitro evidence for an association between steroid hormones and specific fiber components. *Am J Clin Nutr* **51**, 365-70 (1990).

184. Fuchs, C.S. et al. Dietary fiber and the risk of colorectal cancer and adenoma in women. *N Engl J Med* **340**, 169-76 (1999).

185. Reddy, B.S. Role of dietary fiber in colon cancer: an overview. *Am J Med* **106**, 16S-19S; discussion 50S-51S (1999).

186. Honda, T., Kai, I. & Ohi, G. Fat and dietary fiber intake and colon cancer mortality: a chronological comparison between Japan and the United States. *Nutr Cancer* **33**, 95-9 (1999).

187. Terry, P., Jain, M., Miller, A.B., Howe, G.R. & Rohan, T.E. No association among total dietary fiber, fiber fractions, and risk of breast cancer. *Cancer Epidemiol Biomarkers Prev* **11**, 1507-8 (2002).

188. Protein-sparing diets. *Med Lett Drugs Ther* **19**, 69-70 (1977).

189. "Liquid protein diets" and "protein-sparing modified fast". *N Engl J Med* **299**, 419-21 (1978).

190. Use of protein-sparing modified fast in treatment of diabetes and obesity. *J Tenn Med Assoc* **72**, 682-4 (1979).

191. Bell, L., Chan, L. & Pencharz, P.B. Protein-sparing diet for severely obese adolescents: design and use of an equivalency system for menu planning. *J Am Diet Assoc* **85**, 459-64 (1985).

192. Bellows, J.G. & Bellows, R.T. Protein-sparing diet therapy. *Compr Ther* **4**, 3-4 (1978).

193. Bistrian, D.R., Winterer, J., Blackburn, G.L., Young, V. & Sherman, M. Effect of a protein-sparing diet and brief fast on nitrogen metabolism in mildly obese subjects. *J Lab Clin Med* **89**, 1030-5 (1977).

194. Bistrian, B.R., Blackburn, G.L. & Stanbury, J.B. Metabolic aspects of a protein-sparing modified fast in the dietary management of Prader-Willi obesity. *N Engl J Med* **296**, 774-9 (1977).

195. Bistrian, B.R. Clinical use of a protein-sparing modified fast. *Jama* **240**, 2299-302 (1978).

196. Bistrian, B.R. & Sherman, M. Results of the treatment of obesity with a protein-sparing modified fast. *Int J Obes* **2**, 143-8 (1978).

197. Contaldo, F., Di Biase, G., Scalfi, L., Presta, E. & Mancini, M. Protein-sparing modified fast in the treatment of severe obesity: weight loss and nitrogen balance data. *Int J Obes* **4**, 189-96 (1980).

198. Craig, D.W. Treatment of morbid obesity with protein-sparing modified fast. *J Ark Med Soc* **78**, 489-96 (1982).

199. Everse, J.W. Recent developments in protein-sparing therapy. *Hormoner* **12**, 1-14 (1959).

200. Iselin, H.U. & Burckhardt, P. Balanced hypocaloric diet versus protein-sparing modified fast in the treatment of obesity: a comparative study. *Int J Obes* **6**, 175-81 (1982).

201. Jourdan, M., Margen, S. & Bradfield, R.B. Protein-sparing effect in obese women fed low calorie diets. *Am J Clin Nutr* **27**, 3-12 (1974).

202. Seim, H.C. & Rigden, S.R. Approaching the protein-sparing modified fast. *Am Fam Physician* **42**, 51S-56S (1990).

203. Vermeulen, A. Effects of a short-term (4 weeks) protein-sparing modified fast on plasma lipids and lipoproteins in obese women. *Ann Nutr Metab* **34**, 133-42 (1990).

204. Wadden, T.A., Stunkard, A.J., Brownell, K.D. & Day, S.C. A comparison of two very-low-calorie diets: protein-sparing-modified fast versus protein-formula-liquid diet. *Am J Clin Nutr* **41**, 533-9 (1985).

205. Brown, J.M., Yetter, J.F., Spicer, M.J. & Jones, J.D. Cardiac complications of protein-sparing modified fasting. *Jama* **240**, 120-2 (1978).

206. Banting, W. *Letter on corpulence: addressed to the public*, 22 p. (Printed by Harrison and Sons, [London], 1863).

207. Blanchard, G. et al. Rapid weight loss with a high-protein low-energy diet allows the recovery of ideal body composition and insulin sensitivity in obese dogs. *J Nutr* **134**, 2148S-2150S (2004).

208. Donini, L.M., Pinto, A. & Cannella, C. [High-protein diets and obesity]. *Ann Ital Med Int* **19**, 36-42 (2004).

209. Eisenstein, J., Roberts, S.B., Dallal, G. & Saltzman, E. High-protein weight-loss diets: are they safe and do they work? A review of the experimental and epidemiologic data. *Nutr Rev* **60**, 189-200 (2002).

210. Fitz, J.D., Sperling, E.M. & Fein, H.G. A hypocaloric high-protein diet as primary therapy for adults with obesity-related diabetes: effective long-term use in a community hospital. *Diabetes Care* **6**, 328-33 (1983).

211.   Howard, A.N. & Anderson, T.B. The treatment of obesity with a high-protein loaf. *Practitioner* **201**, 491-6 (1968).

212.   Johnston, C.S., Day, C.S. & Swan, P.D. Postprandial thermogenesis is increased 100% on a high-protein, low-fat diet versus a high-carbohydrate, low-fat diet in healthy, young women. *J Am Coll Nutr* **21**, 55-61 (2002).

213.   Korobov, D.M. & Petrosian, A.A. [Experience with a high-protein reducing diet in the treatment of obesity]. *Vopr Pitan* **26**, 62-4 (1967).

214.   Luscombe, N.D., Clifton, P.M., Noakes, M., Farnsworth, E. & Wittert, G. Effect of a high-protein, energy-restricted diet on weight loss and energy expenditure after weight stabilization in hyperinsulinemic subjects. *Int J Obes Relat Metab Disord* **27**, 582-90 (2003).

215.   Robinson, S.M. et al. Protein turnover and thermogenesis in response to high-protein and high-carbohydrate feeding in men. *Am J Clin Nutr* **52**, 72-80 (1990).

216.   Worthington, B.S. & Taylor, L.E. Balanced low-calorie vs. high-protein-low-carbohydrate reducing diets. I. Weight loss, nutrient intake, and subjective evaluation. *J Am Diet Assoc* **64**, 47-51 (1974).

217.   Bowen, J., Noakes, M. & Clifton, P.M. Effect of calcium and dairy foods in high protein, energy-restricted diets on weight loss and metabolic parameters in overweight adults. *Int J Obes Relat Metab Disord* (2005).

218. Clifton, P.M., Noakes, M., Keogh, J. & Foster, P. Effect of an energy reduced high protein red meat diet on weight loss and metabolic parameters in obese women. *Asia Pac J Clin Nutr* **12 Suppl**, S10 (2003).

219. Garcia de los Rios, M., Carrasco, E., Padilla, M., Fonseca, B. & Lopez, G. [Treatment of obesity with a liquid, relatively high protein diet (author's transl)]. *Rev Med Chil* **108**, 691-6 (1980).

220. Halton, T.L. & Hu, F.B. The effects of high protein diets on thermogenesis, satiety and weight loss: a critical review. *J Am Coll Nutr* **23**, 373-85 (2004).

221. Westerterp-Plantenga, M.S., Rolland, V., Wilson, S.A. & Westerterp, K.R. Satiety related to 24 h diet-induced thermogenesis during high protein/carbohydrate vs high fat diets measured in a respiration chamber. *Eur J Clin Nutr* **53**, 495-502 (1999).

222. Westerterp-Plantenga, M.S., Lejeune, M.P., Nijs, I., van Ooijen, M. & Kovacs, E.M. High protein intake sustains weight maintenance after body weight loss in humans. *Int J Obes Relat Metab Disord* **28**, 57-64 (2004).

223. Zed, C. & James, W.P. Dietary thermogenesis in obesity. Response to carbohydrate and protein meals: the effect of beta-adrenergic blockade and semistarvation. *Int J Obes* **10**, 391-405 (1986).

224. Watanabe, A., Wakabayashi, H. & Kuwabara, Y. Nutrient-induced thermogenesis and protein-sparing effect by rapid infusion of a branched chain-enriched amino acid solution to cirrhotic patients. *J Med* **27**, 176-82 (1996).

225. Soucy, J. & Leblanc, J. Protein meals and postprandial thermogenesis. *Physiol Behav* **65**, 705-9 (1999).

226. Schutz, Y., Bray, G. & Margen, S. Postprandial thermogenesis at rest and during exercise in elderly men ingesting two levels of protein. *J Am Coll Nutr* **6**, 497-506 (1987).

227. Garrow, J.S. The contribution of protein synthesis to thermogenesis in man. *Int J Obes* **9 Suppl 2**, 97-101 (1985).

228. Brito, M.N., Botion, L.M., Brito, N.A., Kettelhut, I.C. & Migliorini, R.H. Lipolysis and glycerokinase activity in brown adipose tissue of rat fed a high protein, carbohydrate-free diet. *Horm Metab Res* **26**, 51-2 (1994).

229. Kettelhut, I.C., Foss, M.C. & Migliorini, R.H. Lipolysis and the antilipolytic effect of insulin in adipocytes from rats adapted to a high-protein diet. *Metabolism* **34**, 69-73 (1985).

230. Megia, A. et al. Protein intake during aggressive calorie restriction in obesity determines growth hormone response to growth hormone-releasing hormone after weight loss. *Clin Endocrinol (Oxf)* **39**, 217-20 (1993).

231. Rasmussen, M.H., Juul, A., Kjems, L.L., Skakkebaek, N.E. & Hilsted, J. Lack of stimulation of 24-hour growth hormone release by hypocaloric diet in obesity. *J Clin Endocrinol Metab* **80**, 796-801 (1995).

232. Tanaka, K. et al. Very-low-calorie diet-induced weight reduction reverses impaired growth hormone secretion response to growth hormone-releasing hormone, arginine, and L-dopa in obesity. *Metabolism* **39**, 892-6 (1990).

233. Hara, M. et al. Effects of a low-protein diet on prolactin- and growth hormone-producing cells in the rat pituitary gland. *Anat Rec* **251**, 37-43 (1998).

234. Heffernan, M.A. et al. Increase of fat oxidation and weight loss in obese mice caused by chronic treatment with human growth hormone or a modified C-terminal fragment. *Int J Obes Relat Metab Disord* **25**, 1442-9 (2001).

235. Rasmussen, M.H. et al. Massive weight loss restores 24-hour growth hormone release profiles and serum insulin-like growth factor-I levels in obese subjects. *J Clin Endocrinol Metab* **80**, 1407-15 (1995).

236. Anderson, I.M., Crook, W.S., Gartside, S.E., Fairburn, C.G. & Cowen, P.J. The effect of moderate weight loss on overnight growth hormone and cortisol secretion in healthy female volunteers. *J Affect Disord* **16**, 197-202 (1989).

237. Liu, S. et al. Relation between changes in intakes of dietary fiber and grain products and changes in weight and development of obesity among middle-aged women. *Am J Clin Nutr* **78**, 920-7 (2003).

238. Ebbeling, C.B., Leidig, M.M., Sinclair, K.B., Hangen, J.P. & Ludwig, D.S. A reduced-glycemic load diet in the treatment of adolescent obesity. *Arch Pediatr Adolesc Med* **157**, 773-9 (2003).

239. Meshcheriakova, V.A., Plotnikova, O.A., Sharafetdinov, K. & Iatsyshina, T.A. [The use of the combined food products with soy protein in diet therapy for patients with diabetes mellitus type 2]. *Vopr Pitan* **71**, 19-24 (2002).

240. Stephenson, T.J. et al. Effect of soy protein-rich diet on renal function in young adults with insulin-dependent diabetes mellitus. *Clin Nephrol* **64**, 1-11 (2005).

241. Beilin, L.J., Burke, V., Puddey, I.B., Mori, T.A. & Hodgson, J.M. Recent developments concerning diet and hypertension. *Clin Exp Pharmacol Physiol* **28**, 1078-82 (2001).

242. Endoh, M., Odamaki, M., Ikegaya, N. & Kumagai, H. Factors involved in the development of hypertension induced by a low-protein diet in rats with renal injury. *Kidney Blood Press Res* **27**, 1-9 (2004).

243. Langley-Evans, S.C. Critical differences between two low protein diet protocols in the programming of hypertension in the rat. *Int J Food Sci Nutr* **51**, 11-7 (2000).

244. Langley-Evans, S.C., Welham, S.J. & Jackson, A.A. Fetal exposure to a maternal low protein diet impairs nephrogenesis and promotes hypertension in the rat. *Life Sci* **64**, 965-74 (1999).

245. Langley-Evans, S.C. Hypertension induced by foetal exposure to a maternal low-protein diet, in the rat, is prevented by pharmacological blockade of maternal glucocorticoid synthesis. *J Hypertens* **15**, 537-44 (1997).

246. Dwyer, J.T., Allison, D.B. & Coates, P.M. Dietary supplements in weight reduction. *J Am Diet Assoc* **105**, S80-6 (2005).

247. Egger, G., Cameron-Smith, D. & Stanton, R. The effectiveness of popular, non-prescription weight loss supplements. *Med J Aust* **171**, 604-8 (1999).

248. Saper, R.B., Eisenberg, D.M. & Phillips, R.S. Common dietary supplements for weight loss. *Am Fam Physician* **70**, 1731-8 (2004).

249. Bouchard, N.C., Howland, M.A., Greller, H.A., Hoffman, R.S. & Nelson, L.S. Ischemic stroke associated with use of an ephedra-free dietary supplement containing synephrine. *Mayo Clin Proc* **80**, 541-5 (2005).

250. Lee, M.K., Cheng, B.W., Che, C.T. & Hsieh, D.P. Cytotoxicity assessment of Ma-huang (Ephedra) under different conditions of preparation. *Toxicol Sci* **56**, 424-30 (2000).

251. Maglione, M. et al. Psychiatric effects of ephedra use: an analysis of Food and Drug Administration reports of adverse events. *Am J Psychiatry* **162**, 189-91 (2005).

252. McBride, B.F. et al. Electrocardiographic and hemodynamic effects of a multicomponent dietary supplement containing ephedra and caffeine: a randomized controlled trial. *Jama* **291**, 216-21 (2004).

253. Nelson, R. FDA issues alert on ephedra supplements in the USA. *Lancet* **363**, 135 (2004).

254. Schulman, S. Addressing the potential risks associated with ephedra use: a review of recent efforts. *Public Health Rep* **118**, 487-92 (2003).

255. Shekelle, P. & Hardy, M. Safety and efficacy of ephedra and ephedrine for enhancement of athletic performance, thermogenesis and the treatment of obesity. *Phytomedicine* **9**, 78 (2002).

256.   Shekelle, P.G. et al. Efficacy and safety of ephedra and ephedrine for weight loss and athletic performance: a meta-analysis. *Jama* **289**, 1537-45 (2003).

257.   Soni, M.G., Carabin, I.G., Griffiths, J.C. & Burdock, G.A. Safety of ephedra: lessons learned. *Toxicol Lett* **150**, 97-110 (2004).

258.   High iron stores may predict development of type 2 diabetes. *Bmj* **317**, C (1998).

259.   Blood test may measure women's iron levels to predict diabetes risk. *Health News* **10**, 15 (2004).

260.   Dinneen, S.F. et al. Liver iron stores in patients with non-insulin-dependent diabetes mellitus. *Mayo Clin Proc* **69**, 13-5 (1994).

261.   Fernandez-Real, J.M., Lopez-Bermejo, A. & Ricart, W. Cross-talk between iron metabolism and diabetes. *Diabetes* **51**, 2348-54 (2002).

262.   Hernandez, C., Genesca, J., Ignasi Esteban, J., Garcia, L. & Simo, R. [Relationship between iron stores and diabetes mellitus in patients infected by hepatitis C virus: a case-control study]. *Med Clin (Barc)* **115**, 21-2 (2000).

263.   Jiang, R. et al. Body iron stores in relation to risk of type 2 diabetes in apparently healthy women. *Jama* **291**, 711-7 (2004).

264.   Jiang, R. et al. Dietary iron intake and blood donations in relation to risk of type 2 diabetes in men: a prospective cohort study. *Am J Clin Nutr* **79**, 70-5 (2004).

265. Kar, M. & Chakraborti, A.S. Release of iron from haemoglobin--a possible source of free radicals in diabetes mellitus. *Indian J Exp Biol* **37**, 190-2 (1999).

266. Lane, D.M. Iron stores as a risk factor for diabetes in women. *Jama* **291**, 2428; author reply 2428-9 (2004).

267. Lecube Torello, A., Hernandez Pascual, C. & Simo Canonge, R. [Iron overload in adults and its possible relationship with type 2 diabetes mellitus]. *Med Clin (Barc)* **124**, 158-9; author reply 159 (2005).

268. Lee, D.H., Folsom, A.R. & Jacobs, D.R., Jr. Dietary iron intake and Type 2 diabetes incidence in postmenopausal women: the Iowa Women's Health Study. *Diabetologia* **47**, 185-94 (2004).

269. Ortega Calvo, M. [Iron deposits, diabetes mellitus and case-control design]. *Med Clin (Barc)* **115**, 478-9 (2000).

270. Pavlov, K. & Pisanets, M. On iron metabolism in patients with diabetes. *Folia Med (Plovdiv)* **26**, 24-7 (1984).

271. Pan, C., Lu, J. & Tian, H. [Epidemiology of adult diabetes mellitus in a population of Capital Iron and Steel Company in Beijing]. *Zhonghua Yi Xue Za Zhi* **75**, 409-13, 446 (1995).

272. Perez de Nanclares, G. et al. Excess iron storage in patients with type 2 diabetes unrelated to primary hemochromatosis. *N Engl J Med* **343**, 890-1 (2000).

273. Roblin, X., Chevassus, P., Boudemaghe, T. & Palayodan, A. [Should the insulin resistance associated with hepatic iron

overload be researched during diabetes mellitus type II?].
Diabetes Metab **28**, 335-9 (2002).

274. Roza, A.M. et al. Hydroxyethyl starch deferoxamine, a novel
     iron chelator, delays diabetes in BB rats. *J Lab Clin Med* **123**,
     556-60 (1994).

275. Salonen, J.T., Tuomainen, T.P., Nyyssonen, K., Lakka, H.M. &
     Punnonen, K. Relation between iron stores and non-insulin
     dependent diabetes in men: case-control study. *Bmj* **317**, 727
     (1998).

276. Thomas, M.C., MacIsaac, R.J., Tsalamandris, C. & Jerums, G.
     Elevated iron indices in patients with diabetes. *Diabet Med* **21**,
     798-802 (2004).

277. Tilbrook, L. Cross talk between iron metabolism and diabetes.
     Ann Clin Biochem **41**, 255 (2004).

278. Trotter, W.D. Iron stores as a risk factor for diabetes in women.
     Jama **291**, 2428; author reply 2428-9 (2004).

279. Trzeciak, B. [Blood serum iron levels in patients with diabetes
     mellitus aged 40-60 years]. *Przegl Lek* **40**, 555-8 (1983).

280. Vigano, M., Vergani, A., Trombini, P., Paleari, F. & Piperno,
     A. Insulin resistance influence iron metabolism and hepatic
     steatosis in type II diabetes. *Gastroenterology* **118**, 986-7
     (2000).

281. Wilson, J.G., Lindquist, J.H., Grambow, S.C., Crook, E.D. &
     Maher, J.F. Potential role of increased iron stores in diabetes.
     Am J Med Sci **325**, 332-9 (2003).

282. Zuppinger, K. et al. Increased risk of diabetes mellitus in beta-thalassemia major due to iron overload. *Helv Paediatr Acta* **34**, 197-207 (1979).

283. Bannerman, R.M., Keusch, G., Kreimer-Birnbaum, M., Vance, V.K. & Vaughan, S. Thalassemia intermedia, with iron overload, cardiac failure, diabetes mellitus, hypopituitarism and porphyrinuria. *Am J Med* **42**, 476-86 (1967).

284. Matsui, N. et al. Ingested cocoa can prevent high-fat diet-induced obesity by regulating the expression of genes for fatty acid metabolism. *Nutrition* **21**, 594-601 (2005).

285. Flechtner-Mors, M., Biesalski, H.K., Jenkinson, C.P., Adler, G. & Ditschuneit, H.H. Effects of moderate consumption of white wine on weight loss in overweight and obese subjects. *Int J Obes Relat Metab Disord* **28**, 1420-6 (2004).

286. Greenfield, J.R. et al. Moderate alcohol consumption, dietary fat composition, and abdominal obesity in women: evidence for gene-environment interaction. *J Clin Endocrinol Metab* **88**, 5381-6 (2003).

287. Colditz, G.A. et al. Alcohol intake in relation to diet and obesity in women and men. *Am J Clin Nutr* **54**, 49-55 (1991).

288. Adachi, H., Hirai, Y., Fujiura, Y. & Imaizumi, T. [Effect of alcohol intake on dietary habits and obesity in Japanese middle-aged men]. *Nippon Koshu Eisei Zasshi* **47**, 879-86 (2000).

289. Kornhuber, H.H., Lisson, G. & Suschka-Sauermann, L. Alcohol and obesity: a new look at high blood pressure and stroke. An

epidemiological study in preventive neurology. *Eur Arch Psychiatry Neurol Sci* **234**, 357-62 (1985).

290.   Addolorato, G., Capristo, E., Greco, A.V., Stefanini, G.F. & Gasbarrini, G. Influence of chronic alcohol abuse on body weight and energy metabolism: is excess ethanol consumption a risk factor for obesity or malnutrition? *J Intern Med* **244**, 387-95 (1998).

Notes

Printed in the United States
48596LVS00001BA

9 780976 815075